Health Assessment
DeMYSTiFieD

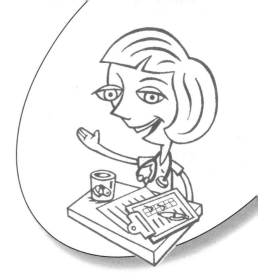

Health Assessment
DeMYSTiFieD

Mary DiGiulio, DNP, RN, ANP-BC
Rutgers, The State University of New Jersey
Bergen Volunteer Medical Initiative

Daria Napierkowski, DNP, RN, ANP-BC, CNE
William Paterson University

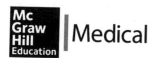 Medical

New York   Chicago   San Francisco   Athens   London   Madrid
Mexico City   Milan   New Delhi   Singapore   Sydney   Toronto

Health Assessment Demystified

1 2 3 4 5 6 7 8 9 0   DOC/DOC   18 17 16 15 14 13

ISBN 978-0-07-177201-3
MHID 0-07-177201-4

This book was set in Berling by Cenveo® Publisher Services.
The editors were Andrew Moyer and Christina M. Thomas.
The production supervisor was Richard Ruzycka.
Project management was provided by Sheena Uprety, Cenveo Publisher Services.
RR Donnelley was the printer and binder.

Library of Congress Cataloging-in-Publication Data

DiGiulio, Mary.
    Health assessment demystified / Mary DiGiulio, RN, MSN, APRN, Daria Napierkowski, DNP, RN, ANP-BC, CNE, William Paterson University.
        pages cm
    Includes index.
        ISBN 978-0-07-177201-3 (pbk.)—ISBN 0-07-177201-4 (pbk.)   1. Nursing diagnosis.
    I. Napierkowski, Daria.   II. Title.
      √RT48.6.D54 2013 4
      616.07′5—dc23
                                                                        2013026976

McGraw-Hill Education books are available at special quantity discounts to use as premiums and sales promotions, or for use in corporate training programs. To contact a representative please e-mail us at bulksales@mcgraw-hill.com.

In memory of Jim, Rose & Margot

—Mary

To my family who supports me and to Jesus Christ who strengthens me

—Daria Napierkowski

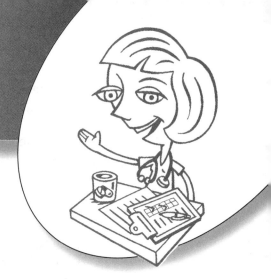

Contents

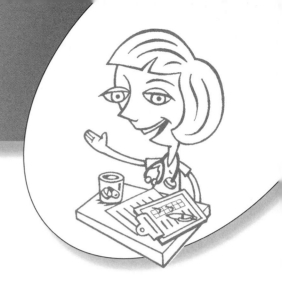

Contributors

Kimberly Buff-Prado, DNP, RN, ANP-BC
Patricia Hindin, PhD, CNM
Frank Manole, DNP, MSN, ACNP-BC
Janet Regan-Livingston, MSN, RN, FNP-C
Susan Wiedaseck, DNP, CNM

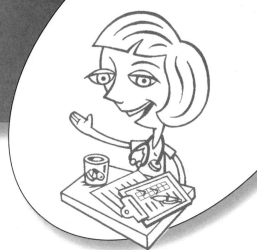

Introduction/Preface

Every healthcare provider needs to be able to correctly identify the signs and symptoms of disease. This book will help you accurately assess each system of the body, ask the appropriate questions, identify risk factors, correctly perform a physical examination, recognize abnormalities, and identify age-related changes.

Health Assessment Demystified contains 17 chapters, with each providing a review of anatomy and physiology of a major body system and a review of common disorders and diseases that can affect that system. Each chapter is divided into the following sections:

- Review of Anatomy and Physiology
- Subjective Information
- Objective Information
- Expected Findings
- Abnormal Findings
- Age-Related Changes
- Cultural Considerations
- Chapter Review Questions and Answers

The anatomy and physiology section includes a review of the structure and function of the major organs of that system. The subjective information section contains questions to ask during the interview process including review of systems (ROS), risk factors related to the system, and risk evaluation. The objective information section states the equipment needed for the physical examination, including the important assessment techniques and how to master them. The expected findings and abnormal findings sections review what the healthcare provider can expect to find in normal and diseased states. Pediatric and geriatric age-related changes are discussed as well as cultural considerations. The chapters conclude with 10 questions and answers to review your knowledge of the system.

A Look Inside

As health assessment can be challenging, this book was written to provide an organized, outlined approach to learn about how to successfully assess body systems and the part the healthcare provider can play in the treatment process.

A thumbnail description of each chapter has been provided in the following.

Chapter 1: Communication Techniques and Collecting Subjective Information

In this chapter, you will learn the important communication skills to become an expert listener and conduct a quality assessment of a patient. It is important for the healthcare provider be a good listener and understand the proper techniques when interviewing a patient. We communicate with our voice and the tone, intensity, and pitch convey important information as well as the actual words that we use. This chapter reviews specific communication skills, including the type of questions to ask the patient, listening skills, and misleading questions to avoid. The nursing process, as well as specific questions to ask the patient concerning a complaint, is reviewed.

Chapter 2: Collecting Objective Information and Documentation

Collecting objective data is important to help identify a correlation between the patient's complaints and the physical examination. Objective data include physical findings discovered by the healthcare provider as well as vital signs, appearance and behavior of the patient, and laboratory data. In this chapter, you will learn the four basic assessment techniques as well as how to correctly document in the patient record. Guidelines for documentation and the healthcare forms one might use are discussed.

Chapter 3: Assessment of Vital Signs

It is important for the healthcare provider to correctly measure the patient's vital signs. In this chapter, the correct techniques of assessing a patient's temperature, pulse, respirations, and blood pressure are discussed. You will learn the normal vital sign ranges from newborn to adult, and the terms used when vital signs are abnormal.

Chapter 4: Assessment of Mental Status

The patient's mental status is assessed throughout the entire interview process and physical examination. In this chapter, you will learn about the nervous system and neurotransmitters and how they relate to the patients mental well-being. A systematic approach to assessing the patient's mental status is discussed including how to assess the patient's alertness, level of orientation, mood, and speech qualities.

Chapter 5: Assessment of the Skin, Hair, and Nails

The assessment of the patient skin, hair, and nails can be performed as an individual assessment or part of the complete physical examination. In this chapter, you will learn about the layers of the skin and the functioning of the skin and its appendages. Important changes that can occur in the skin and how to correctly identify abnormalities such as skin cancer are discussed. You will learn how to correctly document abnormalities assessed on the skin, hair, and nails.

Chapter 6: Assessment of the Head, Eyes, Ears, Nose, and Throat (HEENT)

The head and neck region is important to assess because abnormalities found within this area may reflect disorders of the structures involved or within other body systems. In this chapter, you will review the anatomy and physiology of the head, eyes, ears, nose, mouth, and throat. It is important for the healthcare provider to review this assessment, because it includes the eyes and ears that provide sensory information that help us to safely assess and interact with our environment.

Chapter 7: Assessment of the Respiratory System

The respiratory system assists the body in obtaining oxygen through inhalation and releases carbon dioxide through exhalation. Any change in the respiratory system will affect the oxygenation of all cells within the body. In this chapter, you will learn review of the anatomy and physiology of the respiratory system, gas exchange including normal respiratory rates, and information regarding checking peripheral oxygenation rates. Definitions of abnormal findings are delineated.

Chapter 8: Assessment of the Cardiac and Peripheral Vascular System

The heart contracts to pump blood to the rest of the body. Blood travels from the heart through arteries and returns to the heart through veins. In this chapter, you will review the cardiac anatomy, normal function, cardiac cycle, electrical conduction of the heart, and the best areas to palpate for peripheral pulses. Important associated symptoms are discussed. Abnormal heart sounds and murmurs are defined.

Chapter 9: Assessment of the Abdomen, Pelvis, Anus, and Rectum

Assessment of the abdomen involves several different body systems and complaints of pain in this area can be difficult to distinguish. In this chapter, for assessment purposes you will review the four quadrants and nine subsections of the abdomen. The structure and function of the main organs in each quadrant are discussed. The body mass index and a risk evaluation for abdominal conditions are also reviewed.

Chapter 10: Assessment of the Musculoskeletal System

Can you imagine what the body would be like without the support of the bones and muscles? This chapter will review the structure and function of the bones, joints, and muscles. Skeletal muscle movements are defined to help the healthcare provider perform a functional assessment. Specific tests are important to perform if an abnormality of the joint, bone, or muscle is suspected.

Chapter 11: Assessment of the Nervous System

Most of our bodily functions, both voluntary and involuntary, are controlled through the proper functioning of the nervous system. The nervous system consists of the central nervous system (the brain and spinal cord) and the peripheral nervous system (the nerves that transport impulses to and from the central nervous system). In this chapter, you will learn how to assess the patient's cerebellar and sensory function, 12 cranial nerves, and reflexes through the lifespan of the newborn to adulthood.

Chapter 12: Assessment of the Male Genitourinary System

It is important for the healthcare provider to be comfortable discussing and examining the male genitourinary system. In this chapter, you will learn about the organs involved in reproduction and urination in the male patient. Expected and abnormal findings are stated along with normal age-related changes.

Chapter 13: Assessment of the Female Reproductive System

Assessment of the female reproductive system involves the breasts and genital area. In this chapter, you will learn how to evaluate disorders of the breast and organs of reproduction in the female patient.

Chapter 14: Assessment of the Pregnant Patient

The healthcare provider must be aware of the effects that pregnancy has on the body and be able to differentiate between expected and unexpected changes. In this chapter, you will learn how to assess the normal changes that occur during pregnancy.

Chapter 15: Assessment of Pain

Pain indicates actual or potential injury to the body. It is important for the healthcare provider to successfully assess and treat the patient in pain. In this chapter, you will learn about the different types of pain and common pain theories. Expected findings related to the different types of pain are stated.

Chapter 16: The Head to Toe Comprehensive Assessment

In this chapter, you will learn how to put all assessments together in an organized manner. Important interview questions are discussed including the review of systems presented in a head to toe fashion and how to perform a complete comprehensive assessment in an efficient approach.

Chapter 17: Comprehensive Review Questions

This chapter provides 100 questions and answers to help you review all that you have learnt to be successful in completing a comprehensive health assessment.

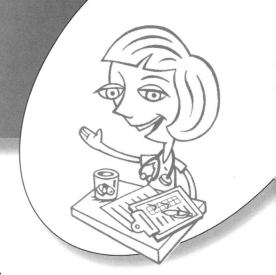

About the Authors

Mary DiGiulio is an adult nurse practitioner, currently on the faculty of the School of Nursing at Rutgers, the State University of New Jersey, and practices at Bergen Volunteer Medical Initiative in Hackensack, NJ. She has taught in various programs of nursing including practical nursing (PN), baccalaureate (BSN), traditional and accelerated RN to BSN, graduate (MSN), and doctoral-level (DNP) students. She has developed and presented review content for Nurse Practitioner, RN, and PN review courses and nurse refresher courses. She has presented at local, regional, national, and international conferences.

Daria Napierkowski is an adult nurse practitioner on the faculty of the School of Nursing at William Paterson University in Wayne, NJ, and practices at the Health and Wellness Center on the campus. She has taught all levels of nursing including the licensed practical nurse, prelicensed programs; accelerated and undergraduate, graduate, and doctoral levels. She has presented review courses for medical-surgical nursing as well as critical care nursing certification. She codeveloped a preprogram for academic success for accelerated baccalaureate nursing students and has presented research on this program nationally and internationally.

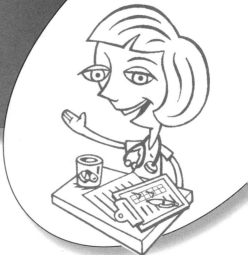

chapter 1

Communication Techniques and Collecting Subjective Information

LEARNING OBJECTIVES

After reviewing this chapter, the learner will be able to:

1 Discuss the qualities of therapeutic communication skills.

2 Determine nonverbal skills used in therapeutic communication.

3 Discuss specific communication skills used in history taking.

4 State the Nursing process.

5 List the four types of assessment.

Communication Skills

The healthcare provider must be an expert in communication skills to conduct a good quality assessment that will reveal the true health status of the patient. The main objective in obtaining the data about the patient is to reveal the patient's health status, lifestyle, nutritional state, cultural preferences, and emotional support available to the patient. The healthcare provider is an advocate for the patient and must first confront personal biases in order to care for all patients of different lifestyles. The healthcare provider should possess expert nonverbal and verbal communication skills.

Nonverbal communication skills include knowing the patient's personal space, touch, and eye contact preferences. The healthcare provider must assess the patient's response to personal touch and how close to be to the patient during the initial history interview. Most patients would prefer the healthcare provider to be about 3-4 ft away with moderate eye contact. Always ask the patient if you can touch them before attempting contact especially during the first meeting with the patient. The healthcare provider's body gestures and posture can show dominance and they should avoid standing over the patient during the interview. Therefore, sit at eye level with the patient and avoid excessive facial and body gestures that might portray annoyance or disinterest.

We communicate with our voices and the tone, intensity, and pitch can convey more information than words. It is important to portray a tone of voice that conveys warmth and confidence using facilitation comments such as: uh huh, go on, continue, etc, to demonstrate your interest in the conversation. Allow for periods of silence and do not hurry the patient as they gather their thoughts to adequately describe their health condition. If the patient is crying, sit with the patient and offer a touch on a shoulder or hold the patient's hand. Ask the patient if he/she would prefer you to continue at a later time. Avoid false reassurance, for example, "don't worry everything will be ok." Such a statement would show lack of interest in the patient, in turn belittling the patient's problems. It is important to be able to realize emotional cues that the patient is exhibiting to develop a relationship of confidence and concern.

Specific Communication Skills

Listening

Listening is one of the most important skills for the healthcare provider to acquire. Be comfortably seated about 3 ft away from the patient and maintain a moderate amount of eye contact and avoid interrupting the patient. You may want to nod or state words of facilitation to ensure the continuation of the conversation. The healthcare provider should keep note-taking to the minimum and avoid facial grimacing or excessive smiling.

Silence

The healthcare provider should avoid trying to fill all lapses in conversation with words, but instead should let the patient gather thoughts in periods of silence. Do not rush the patient, but allow the patient time to contemplate all answers. When the patient is crying, offer comfort by holding the hand or waiting patiently for the patient to compose their thoughts.

Open-Ended Questions

Ask the patient specific question that will allow the patient to discuss symptoms or their medical condition. A typical open-ended question is "How are you feeling today?" or "Tell me about your pain symptoms."

Closed-Ended questions

A closed-ended question requires a one- or two-word response from the patient and does not lead to a discussion. An example is "How old are you?" or "Is there cancer in your family?" A closed-ended question requires a yes or no response.

Giving Examples

Sometimes the patient cannot formulate specific words about a complaint or a symptom. In such circumstances, the healthcare provider needs to provide words to help continue the conversation or obtain detailed information about a symptom. For example, "Is the pain sharp or dull or is it constant or intermittent?"

Continuing the Conversation

The progress of conversation can be facilitated by using specific phrases to continue the conversation without rushing the patient. For example, "Please go on."

Avoiding Misleading Questions

The healthcare provider must avoid adding words or questions to the conversation misleading the patient. For example, "You do not smoke cigarettes, do you?" or "Have you finally quit drinking beer?" This type of questioning may embarrass the patient and will not result in developing a trusting relationship with the patient.

Nursing Process

The purpose of the initial history is to obtain information to develop a plan for the patient. The nursing process is a problem solving tool to develop a plan of care for the patient.

Assessment	The collection process of subjective and objective data.
Diagnosis	The development of a nursing diagnosis based on the subjective and objective data obtained.
Planning	The development of a plan for the patient, with long- and short-term goals that the patient and/or family mutually accept.
Intervention	The implementation of the plan.
Evaluation	The evaluation of the plan involves assessing which interventions were successful and which were not. The healthcare provider returns to the assessment process as needed to update the diagnosis and plan as indicated to help the patient progress to the best health status.

Subjective Data

Collection of subjective and objective data occurs during the assessment of the patient. Subjective data are everything the patient or the patient's family states: health problems, symptom complaints, perceptions of illness, and feelings about disease and illness.

Determine the reason the patient is seeking healthcare. Is there a specific complaint (such as a sore throat), a chronic condition (such as diabetes) in need of follow-up, or are they seeking wellness (preventive) care?

Once the reason for the encounter has been established, determine the necessary information about the complaint, chronic illness, or what prompted the preventive care.

ALERT

The mnemonic PQRST can help the healthcare provider remember specific questions to ask the client about a specific complaint.

For example: The patient complains of abdominal pain.

P: What is the place (location) of the pain? What provokes the abdominal pain? When did the pain start and what were you doing when the pain started?

Q: Tell me the qualities of your pain. Is it sharp, dull, throbbing, gnawing, or achy?

R: Does the pain radiate to another area of your body? Point to the area(s) of pain. Does anything relieve the pain?

S: What is the severity of the pain? How would you rate your pain on a scale of 1-10 with 1 being no pain and 10 being severe pain? Are there any symptoms associated with the pain? For example, nausea, vomiting, constipation, or diarrhea? What is the setting for the pain? For example, does the abdominal pain only occur after eating fatty foods?

T: What is the timing of the pain? Is the pain continuous or intermittent? What makes the pain worse or better? Have you tried any treatments for the pain? Which treatments were successful and which were not helpful?

The healthcare provider will also ask subjective questions regarding:

Past history: All medical illnesses and surgeries the patient has experienced. Treatment for current conditions is included in the past history assessment and complications from surgery.

Medications: What current medication is the patient taking, including the name of the medication, route, dosage, and the time taken? Include all over-the-counter (OTC) medications, vitamins, and herbal preparations.

Childhood illnesses and vaccines: List all childhood illnesses the patient has experienced and avoid documenting usual childhood diseases (UCHDs). Accurate documentation should state: no history of measles, mumps, chickenpox, polio, meningitis, viruses, and otitis media. List all vaccines the patient has received including influenza and pneumonia vaccines. Ask the patient about tuberculosis testing and immunizations received related to travel.

Social history: The social history includes questions concerning the patient's environment, socioeconomics, personal habits, self-care behaviors, occupation, religious and cultural preferences, sexuality, and access to medical care.

Family history: The family history includes the diseases in the patient's immediate family, including the age of onset of illness and the age at death of the mother, father, and siblings, if deceased.

Perception of current state of health: The patient's perception of current health is how the patient perceives the current illness and how the illness is impacting their lifestyle: activities of living (ADLs) and independent activities of living (IADLs), for example, shopping and preparing food.

Types of Assessment

Comprehensive Assessment

Comprehensive assessment includes a complete history and physical examination of the patient. It includes:

1. Current health problems and reason for seeking care.
2. Past medical history: surgeries, accidents, hospitalizations, childhood illness, and allergies.
3. Family history: immediate family history of common diseases.
4. Lifestyle: cigarette smoking, alcohol usage, illicit drug usage, exercise habits, nutritional intake, stress relief, functional ability, religious and cultural preferences.
5. Review of Systems (ROS): questions related to symptoms in each body system in a head to toe fashion.
6. Complete physical examination.

Follow-Up Assessment

Assessment after a health problem has been identified with review of present concerns and identification of any new concerns. It establishes a diagnosis in need of follow-up care.

Focused Assessment

The patient has a specific health problem that needs immediate attention. It is commonly performed after the initial comprehensive assessment has been established.

Emergency Assessment

A rapid assessment is performed when the patient is at risk of death or serious physiologic problems due to the current health problem, and measures are initiated to save the patient's life or prevent further injury.

Review of Systems

The purpose of the review of systems (ROS) is to review past and present complaints of each body system with the patient. The patient is asked specific questions about each body system. Problems addressed include questions about past symptoms and if the complaint is continuing or resolved. The ROS only includes subjective data supplied by the patient or the patient's family and not objective information obtained during the physical examination. Information is often forgotten by the patient until they are asked about a specific complaint. The question is stated in simple terms that the patient can understand, but when documented it is recorded in proper medical terminology being careful to only use approved medical abbreviations. In each chapter, the specific questions the healthcare provider should ask are listed under ROS.

Age-Related Changes

In each chapter, age-related changes are addressed describing the specific developmental changes expected in the pediatric patient and the older adult. Expected and pathologic aging changes are discussed within each specific body system with alterations that are noteworthy.

The approach to and interaction with a young child is different than with the child's parent or grandparent. Care needs to be taken to avoid frightening the patient when dealing with young children. Older patients often need longer time to formulate responses to questions and may experience some difficulty hearing the questions.

Case Study

In each chapter, a case study of the topic identified will be presented and 10 questions related to the chapter will be offered. Explanations of the correct answer will be provided.

REVIEW QUESTIONS

1. **Why is it important to have good communication skills when interviewing patients?**
   A. To obtain accurate data that reveals the patient's health status.
   B. To avoid insulting the patient by sitting too close.
   C. To help the healthcare provider to make an accurate medical diagnosis.
   D. To avoid placing inaccurate information on the medical record.

2. **When is a focused assessment performed?**
   A. When the patient is at risk of dying and life-saving measures are initiated.
   B. When a complete history and physical examination is needed.
   C. After a health problem is identified and new concerns are discussed.
   D. To address specific health problems that require immediate attention.

3. **At which phase of the nursing process does the healthcare provider discuss goals that the patient agrees are important?**
   A. Assessment
   B. Planning
   C. Implementation
   D. Evaluation

4. **When performing the ROS, it is important to remember:**
   A. to include objective data in the medical record.
   B. ask the patient questions in easy to understand language.
   C. to obtain a family history of some complaints.
   D. ask closed-ended questions to obtain accurate information.

5. **Which of the following is an example of an open-ended question?**
   A. How old are you?
   B. Do you have pain in your arm?
   C. In which year did you have the abdominal surgery?
   D. How are you feeling today?

6. **Why is it important to facilitate the conversation when interviewing a patient?**
   A. To obtain accurate responses from the patient.
   B. To indicate an interest in the conversation.
   C. To allow the patient to gather their thoughts.
   D. To avoid misleading the patient.

7. **The problem solving tool the healthcare provider uses to develop a plan of care with the patient is called:**
   A. Initial Comprehensive Assessment.
   B. Nursing process.
   C. ROS.
   D. Intuition.

8. **Which of the following reflects the most accurate method of documenting childhood diseases?**

   A. History of UCHDs.

   B. Patient had an appendectomy at the age of 10 years.

   C. No known history of any childhood illness.

   D. Denies history of measles, mumps, and chickenpox.

9. **What is an important question/statement to ask the patient when assessing medication usage?**

   A. "Are you still taking the same medications?"

   B. "What is the generic name of the medication?"

   C. "Are you using any herbal preparations?"

   D. "I do not need to know if you are taking any OTC medications."

10. **The patient's use of tobacco products is documented in which area of the subjective assessment?**

    A. Perception of illness

    B. Review of Systems (ROS)

    C. Social history

    D. Emergency assessment

ANSWERS

1. A. It is important to have good communication skills to obtain accurate data regarding the patient's current health status. Answer B addresses the patient's comfort level and the provider should sit about 3 ft away from the patient. Answers C and D are important to collect data but do not answer the question about communication skills.

2. D. The focused assessment addressed specific health problems that need immediate attention. An emergency assessment is performed when the patient is at risk of death and actions are initiated to prevent serious consequences to the patient, and when the patient is stable then additional information can be obtained. A complete history and physical examination is considered a comprehensive assessment. A follow-up assessment is performed after a health problem has been identified and any new or present concerns are addressed.

3. B. Planning is when the patient and the provider discuss short- and long-term goals that are mutually agreed upon. Assessment is when subjective and objective data are collected. Implementation is initiating the plan. Evaluation is when the patient and the healthcare provider discuss if the plan was successful. The healthcare provider returns to step one (answer A)—assessment, if the plan was not successful.

4. B. Ask the patient questions in language the patient understands but document in proper medical terminology in the medical record. Objective data and family history are not included in the ROS. Open-ended questions assist in obtaining the ROS to obtain accurate patient symptoms.

5. D. Ask how the patient feels to begin the conversation and to discuss symptoms the patient is experiencing. The other answers (A, B, and C) need a one- or two-word answer and do not stimulate conversation.

6. B. Facilitate the conversation by saying go on or nodding the head to show an interest in the conversation. Silence is used to help the patient gather thoughts. The patient can be misled by asking imposing questions, eg, "Did you quit smoking yet?" It is important to obtain accurate information from the patient but facilitation does not guarantee it.

7. B. The nursing process is a problem solving tool used to develop a plan of care for the patient. The initial comprehensive assessment is used to collect subjective and objective data and is usually performed in the first meeting with the patient. The ROS is a list of questions to ask to obtain information about symptoms of a specific body system. Intuition is knowledge obtained by learning about the disease process and by experience of taking care of patients with specific illnesses, and a "sense" of what may happen next when the patient is experiencing symptoms.

8. D. It is more accurate to state the specific diseases the patient had or denied having as a child. An appendectomy is a surgical procedure and is not a childhood illness.

9. B. It is important to know if the patient is taking any herbal preparations as well as OTC medications. The patient may not be aware of the generic name of the medication and it is important for the healthcare worker to review the name, dosage, route, and time when the medications are taken.

10. C. The social history is where the healthcare provider will document the patient's habits: tobacco, alcohol, illicit drug use, exercise, and diet patterns.

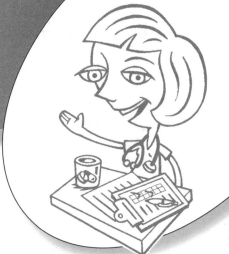

chapter **2**

Collecting Objective Information and Documentation

After reviewing this chapter, the learner will be able to:

❶ Discuss the importance of documentation in the medical record.

❷ Discuss the four types of assessment techniques used in collecting objective data.

❸ State the sounds generated by percussion.

❹ Discuss the guidelines of documentation.

KEYWORDS

Auscultation	Inspection
Documentation	Palpation
Dullness	Percussion
Flatness	Resonance
Hyperresonance	Tympany

Collecting Objective Information

Objective data include all the data collected from the physical examination including: vital signs, appearance, behavior, physical findings, and laboratory testing. Objective data are direct observation and measurement against an accepted standard and are obtained by the four assessment techniques: inspection, palpation, percussion, and auscultation.

Inspection

The healthcare provider inspects the patient by visualizing all the areas while taking time to look at all the systems thoroughly. The senses of smell and hearing are also utilized to note abnormal odors or sounds. It is important to inspect and observe before palpation. With inspection, the healthcare provider should note the following characteristics of the patient: color, pattern, location, size, symmetry, odor, sound, or movement, and compare the symmetry of the body parts. The environment can make a difference with the inspection. Ensuring that the room is a comfortable temperature for the patient will provide a better assessment of the skin, and using good lighting, preferably natural sunlight, will enable better accuracy of the inspection.

Palpation

The healthcare provider utilizes the: dorsal, ulnar/palmar surface, and finger pads of the hand for palpation. The examiner's hand should be at a comfortable temperature and the fingernails should be short, smooth, and trimmed. The ideal parts of the hand to palpate and assess the patient are:

1. Temperature (cold/warm) and moisture (wet/dry) using the dorsal surface of the hand.
2. Vibrations using the palmar surface of the hand.

3. Texture (rough/smooth), mobility (fixed/movable), consistency (soft/hard/fluid filled), strength (weak, thready/strong/bounding of pulses), size (small/medium/large), and shape (irregular/well defined) of masses or degree of tenderness by using the finger pads of the hand.

Even though the depth and thickness of the amount overlying the structure will determine the degree of palpation, the practitioner should first initiate with light palpation before proceeding to moderate, and then to deep palpation.

Light palpation: To assess skin surface, temperature, moisture, tenderness, and pulses. Press with the dominant hand lightly, less than 1 cm, in a slow circular motion.

Moderate palpation: Depressing the skin surface 1-2 cm/0.5-0.75 inch in a slow circular motion to palpate and assess the size, mobility, and consistency of the structure, masses, and body organs.

Deep palpation: Press between 2.5 cm and 5 cm/1-2 inches, using one hand on top of the other, pressing slowly to assess deep structures that are covered by muscle.

Bimanual palpation: Placing the body part in-between two hands. One hand is used to hold and apply pressure, while the other feels the body structure (eg, breast, spleen, uterus) assessing the size and shape of masses.

Percussion

Percussion is the art of tapping either directly against the skin (used in sinus percussion) or against the distal joint of a finger placed on the skin over the anatomic area to be assessed (used in abdominal or thoracic percussion) to elicit: the density of an organ or mass; pain or tenderness from underlying inflammation; size of a mass or organ; or to elicit reflexes. Deep tendon reflexes can be elicited by striking a reflex hammer over a tendon to cause a response.

Sounds Generated by Percussion
Resonance—heard over lung tissue.
Hyperresonance—heard over lung tissue overinflated with air (eg, emphysema).
Tympany—heard over air-filled viscera (eg, abdomen).
Dullness—heard over a dense organ (eg, liver).
Flatness—heard over very dense tissue (eg, bone).

Direct, blunt, and indirect are the three types of percussion utilized.

Direct percussion is the use of one to two finger tips tapping directly over the body part to elicit tenderness, used mainly for eliciting tenderness of the sinuses.

Blunt percussion is performed by one hand flat on the body surface, while the other hand, in a fist, strikes the back of the hand flat on the body surface to elicit tenderness over an organ.

Indirect or mediate percussion is most commonly utilized. This method is used to assess the density of the underlying structures and is performed by using quick sharp taps of the dominant hand's middle finger over the nondominant hand which is resting upon the body part. The composition (solid/fluid/air) of the density of the underlying structure will determine the intensity/loudness and pitch of the sound. As the density increases the intensity of the sound softens, that is, solid tissue elicits a soft tone; the sound increases in intensity/loudness with fluid and air creating the strongest intensity/loudest sound.

Auscultation

Auscultation is a method of using a stethoscope to listen to sounds that are classified to assess for intensity, pitch, quality, and duration of the sound. The diaphragm is used for high-pitched sounds (eg, breath sounds) and the bell is used for low-pitched sounds (eg, murmurs) and abnormal heart sounds (eg, S3 or S4 and bruits).

To get the best outcome of your assessment, listen in a quiet room. Press the diaphragm of the stethoscope firmly and directly to the skin (avoid over clothing as this may obscure the sound) of the body part to listen for high-pitch sounds (ie, breath sounds, bowel sounds, and normal heart sounds). Utilize the bell of the stethoscope for either bruits or abnormal heart sounds (Figure 2-1).

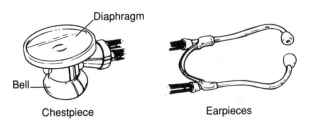

FIGURE 2-1 • Diagram of a stethoscope.
(Reproduced with permission from LeBlond RF, *DeGowin RL, Brown DD: DeGowin's Diagnostic Examination,* 9th edition. New York, NY: McGraw-Hill; 2008. Figure 3-2.)

After obtaining the patient's history, the objective data are obtained through physical examination. The examination of the patient includes: inspection, palpation, percussion, and auscultation. The examination further assesses the patient's problem by validating or invalidating the subjective data obtained.

Methods of validating the data include: clarifying the information with the patient, repeat assessment, and/or verifying the information with a more experienced colleague.

Documentation

Documentation is a valuable tool for communication between the healthcare provider and the other members of the healthcare team involved in the patient's care. The documentation should provide detailed information regarding the evaluation and intervention of the patient's outcome.

Accurate and complete detailed documentation can provide evidence that the healthcare provider was accountable, provided competent and safe care in a timely manner, and practiced within the accepted standards of care. It is a legal document providing support for reimbursement of services and can be used for epidemiologic data for research.

ALERT

Guidelines for Documentation
- Use only approved abbreviations.
- Document objectively without judgmental adjectives.
- Describe what you observe and avoid the word "normal."
- Use descriptive words to describe the patient and avoid wordiness and redundancy.
- Write legibly and neatly using correct grammar and avoid personal opinions.
- Never erase or white-out a word. Instead, draw one line through the word and write "mistake in entry" and write the correct word.
- All complaints by the patient must be documented in the objective portion of the record. For example, subjective data: patient complains of abdominal pain after eating; objective data: pain upon light palpation of right upper quadrant.

- Use of the words "states" or "denies" are more credible. For example, patient states that he/she has pain upon inspiration or patient denies pain upon inspiration.
- Document the patient's expressions of concern about his condition or illness. For example, Mr Jones stated "he is worried he will suffer like his brother did when he was diagnosed with cancer."
- It is not necessary to record how the data were obtained.
- At the end of the objective examination, review all subjective and objective data for missing data and repeat parts of the assessment as needed.

Forms Used to Document

Each institution of healthcare has unique forms to document patient illness and progress. Standardized forms must meet criteria of certifying agencies as well as government and insurance reimbursement standards. There are many types of assessment forms used to document data in the patient's record. An open-ended form includes a narrative story of the patient's illness or disease and is timed and dated with updates as necessary. This type of form takes a significant amount of time to complete. A checklist type of form will have standardized language of data and the healthcare provider will place a check in the correct box that demonstrates the patient's current condition. There is usually a comment section for additional data the provider would like to add for further clarification of the patient's current state of illness. Most institutions are using computers to document data and the healthcare provider will be provided training to learn how to use the computer documentation forms. Documentation on the computer needs to be as accurate as data on paper and usually requires a password to protect the privacy of the patient.

REVIEW QUESTIONS

1. **The sound generated by tapping on the chest wall over normal lung tissue is called?**
   A. Percussion
   B. Tympany
   C. Resonance
   D. Dullness

2. **During light palpation, the fingers are depressed:**

    A. greater than 1 cm.

    B. about 2-5 cm.

    C. 1 cm or less.

    D. greater than 5 cm.

3. **During the inspection phase of an objective assessment, it is important to:**

    A. perform inspection quickly to expedite the examination.

    B. determine the texture of the skin.

    C. note abnormal sounds or odors.

    D. use the diaphragm of the stethoscope.

4. **The most commonly used method of percussion is:**

    A. direct.

    B. blunt.

    C. indirect.

    D. bimanual.

5. **The healthcare provider is utilizing percussion and understands that _____ creates the strongest intensity or loudest tone?**

    A. Air

    B. Fluid

    C. Solid

    D. Mass

6. **Which of the following is *not* a method of palpation?**

    A. Light

    B. Moderate

    C. Deep

    D. Blunt

    E. Bimanual

7. **Which of the following *best* describes moderate palpation?**

    A. Nondominant hand depressing the skin 1-2 cm, in a rectangular motion.

    B. Dominant hand depressing the skin less than 1 cm, in a slow rectangular motion.

    C. Dominant hand depressing the skin 1-2 cm, in a slow circular motion.

    D. Using both hands, one on each side of the body part.

8. The diaphragm of the stethoscope is used to auscultate which of the following types of sounds? *Select all that apply.*

   A. High pitched
   B. Normal heart sounds
   C. Breath sounds
   D. Abnormal heart sounds and bruits

9. What is obtained from the physical examination?

   A. Patient's complaints of pain.
   B. Tenderness elicited over an area.
   C. Patient's date of birth.
   D. History of surgeries.

10. It is important for the healthcare provider to avoid documenting personal opinions about the patient because:

   A. the patient will sue the provider.
   B. it avoids personal bias.
   C. it is required by all institutions.
   D. it avoids redundancy.

ANSWERS

1. C. Resonance is the sound generated when percussing (tapping) over normal lung tissue. Tympany is the sound generated over air-filled viscera (eg, abdomen). Dullness is the sound generated over a dense organ (eg, liver).

2. C. During light palpation, the fingers are depressed no greater than 1 cm or less. During deep palpation, the fingers are depressed 2.5-5 cm.

3. C. During the inspection phase of the assessment, take the time to look, listen, and smell. It should not be done in a hurry. Palpation is a method used to determine texture of the skin and auscultation is a method that uses a stethoscope to listen to sounds generated by the body.

4. C. The most commonly used method of percussion is indirect or mediate percussion.

5. A. Air. As the density increases, the intensity of a sound softens. Thus, air would create the loudest sound/tone.

6. D. All are methods of palpation, except that "blunt" is a method used in percussion not in palpation.

7. C. Moderate palpation entails depressing the skin with the dominant hand 1-2 cm, in a slow circular motion, assessing for body organs/masses. Light palpation is the use of the dominant hand on the surface of the structure depressing less than 1 cm, whereas deep palpation is depressing the surface 2.5-5 cm to assess for deep organs covered by muscle using a technique of the dominant hand on the skin with the nondominant hand on top to apply pressure. Bimanual palpation requires both the hands, one on each side of the body part.

8. A, B, C. The bell of the stethoscope is utilized to auscultate abnormal heart sounds and bruits.

9. B. The examiner must perform the objective examination and can elicit pain or tenderness by palpation over body areas. The other answers are stated in the subjective examination.

10. B. The healthcare provider should not document personal opinions about the patient to avoid personal bias and judgment of the patient.

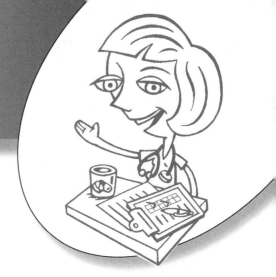

chapter 3

Assessment of Vital Signs

LEARNING OBJECTIVES

After reviewing this chapter, the learner will be able to:

1 Discuss the importance of taking a patient's vital signs.

2 Describe the five methods of taking a patient's temperature.

3 Discuss the proper technique to take a patient's pulse.

4 Apply the correct technique to take a blood pressure.

5 State the stages of blood pressure.

6 Define the orthostatic changes in blood pressure.

Introduction

The healthcare provider is assessing the patient from the beginning of their first encounter until the end of the physical examination. The healthcare provider observes the patient's physical appearance, manner of dress, hygiene, and posture. The healthcare provider notes if the mental condition of the patient is appropriate to the patient situation. The healthcare provider starts the physical examination by taking the vital signs of the patient. It is important to have baseline vital signs to compare with the current vital signs. The proper procedure for checking the temperature followed by pulse, respirations, and blood pressure will be discussed.

Temperature

The average temperature taken by an oral thermometer is 98.6°F (37°C). The patient's temperature in the early morning is lower than average and is higher than average in the late afternoon or evening. The rectal temperature is higher than the oral temperature by about 1°F. The axillary temperature is usually lower than the oral and rectal temperature by about 1°F and can take up to 10 minutes to register. The tympanic and temporal temperature is higher than the average oral temperature by about 1°F. A patient's temperature can range from 96.7°F (35.9°C) to 100°F (37.8°C) depending on the method used to take the temperature and time of day the healthcare provider takes the temperature of the patient. The temperature will also fluctuate with exercise, pregnancy, menstrual cycle, emotional stress, age, gender, and the patient's state of physical health.

It is important for the healthcare provider to remember that it is his/her responsibility to check to ensure that all equipment is working properly. If the task of checking vital signs is delegated to other personnel, it is important to ensure that they have been properly trained in the correct procedures to take vital signs.

Oral Temperature Technique

The average range of the patient's temperature taken by the oral method is 96.4°F-99.1°F (36.8°C-37.3°C). The patient needs to be alert and capable of holding the thermometer in a closed mouth. The healthcare provider should wait 30 minutes if the patient has had a hot or cold beverage to drink or has recently smoked a cigarette. The healthcare provider should place the oral probe under the patient's tongue in the sublingual pocket. This area under the tongue has a good blood supply. This method cannot be used for a patient who is in an unconscious state or is incapable of holding the thermometer in their mouth due to oral trauma or oral surgery. It is not recommended to take an oral temperature on a child under the age of 7 years.

Axillary Temperature Technique

The average range of a patient's temperature taken by the axillary method is 95.9°F-98.6°F (35.5°C-37°C). The axillary method measures surface skin temperature and is the least reliable method, but is commonly used in infants and young children.

Rectal Temperature Technique

The average range of the patient's temperature taken by the rectal method is 97.1°F-100.4°F (36.2°C-38.0°C). This method has been commonly used in the past and reflects the core temperature of the body. However, it is now considered an invasive procedure and is not recommended for infants and small children or for those patients with diarrhea, rectal surgery, lesions of the rectal area, and for the immunocompromised patient The healthcare provider should don gloves and apply a water-soluble lubricant to the rectal probe. The healthcare provider should insert the rectal probe no deeper than 1 inch into the adult rectum.

Tympanic Temperature Technique

The average range of the patient's temperature taken by the tympanic method is 95.7°F-100.0°F (35.4°C-37.8°C). The tympanic membrane probe is inserted about 0.5 cm into the ear canal and the temperature of the tympanic membrane is measured. If performed properly, it is an effective and quick method to take the patient's temperature. This method can be used with a patient who is unconscious or in an acute emergency situation. This temperature is not affected by smoking or oral intake, but should not be used with the patient with ear pain or an ear infection.

Temporal Temperature Technique

The average range of the patient's temperature taken by the temporal method is 98.7°F-100.5°F (37.1°C-38.1°C). This method is a quick and easy way to take the patient's temperature and it measures the heat from the temporal artery. It is suggested that the patient does not have any facial lotion on the forehead and that the thermometer is not swiped too quickly across the forehead. The infrared lens of the thermometer must be kept clean of the skin's oil. This technique can be used with patients in most circumstances and should not be used if there is trauma to the forehead or face.

Definitions	
Hypothermia	Temperature below average range.
Hyperthermia	Temperature above average range.
Bradycardia	Heart rate less than 60 beats per minute.
Tachycardia	Heart rate greater than 100 beats per minute.
Sinus arrhythmia	Heart rhythm increases with inspiration and decreases with expiration, and is common in children and young adults.
Pulse deficit	Difference between a peripheral pulse and apical pulse.
Eupnea	Within normal range of breathing
Tachypnea	Breathing more frequently than normal (more than 20 breaths per minute in the adult).
Bradypnea	Breathing less frequently than normal (less than 12 breaths per minute in the adult).
Dyspnea	Difficulty with breathing.
Orthopnea	Difficulty with breathing in the supine position, prompting the need to sit up to breathe.

Pulse

The pulses are generated when the left ventricle pumps blood into the aorta and generates a pressure wave. The pulse can be felt over a peripheral artery and also at the apical impulse at the fifth intercostal space, at the midclavicular line on the left side (apex of the heart).

TABLE 3-1 Normal Pulse Rate Levels		
Stage	**Age Range**	**Pulse Rate, Beats per Minute**
Newborn	Birth to 3 mo	100-150
Infant	3-6 mo	90-120
	6-12 mo	80-120
Toddler	1-3 y	70-150
Preschooler	3-6 y	70-130
School-aged child	6-12 y	65-125
Adolescent and adult	Over 12 y	60-100
Conditioned athlete	Over 12 y	40-60

The heart rate is defined as the number of pulsations (beats) counted within 1 minute. The healthcare provider assesses the pulse for rate, rhythm, amplitude, and elasticity of the pulse. The average heart rate is 60-100 beats per minute in an adult. The average heart rate varies with age, gender, exercise, pain, medications, stress, and disease state. A well-conditioned athlete can have a heart rate between 40 and 60 beats per minute (see Table 3-1). The rhythm of the pulse can be regular or irregular. A regular pulse is evenly spaced between beats and the irregular pulse is unevenly spaced between beats. The amplitude of the pulse is defined as the ease with which the pulse can be obliterated (see Table 3-2). The elasticity of the pulse is the resilience of the artery. A pulse deficit is the difference between an apical pulse and a peripheral pulse.

Technique

The healthcare provider takes the radial pulse using the pads of the fingers at the lateral aspect of the anterior wrist. If the pulse is regular in rhythm, the

TABLE 3-2 Amplitude of Pulse	
Amplitude of Pulse	
0	Nonpalable pulse or no pulse
1+	Weak, thready pulse and easily obliterated
2+	Normal pulse, felt with a moderate amount of pressure
3+	Bounding, easily felt and difficult to obliterate

healthcare provider can take the pulse for 30 seconds and multiply by two. If the pulse is irregular, the healthcare provider should take the radial pulse for one full minute. The apical pulse should be taken for one full minute, listening for changes in rate, rhythm, and heart sounds. The other places where the healthcare provider can palpate the pulses are not commonly counted but assessed for pulse amplitude and compared bilaterally.

These areas are:

Head and Neck

Temporal artery: In the temple area, anterior to the natural hairline by the top of the ear.

Carotid artery: In the space between the sternomastoid muscle and the trachea.

Arm

Brachial: About 0.5 inch above the antecubital fossa of the elbow, medial side.

Radial: Medial to the radius bone on dorsal side of the hand turned upward, proximal to the thumb.

Ulnar: Medial on the wrist with the palm turned upward (see Figure 3-1).

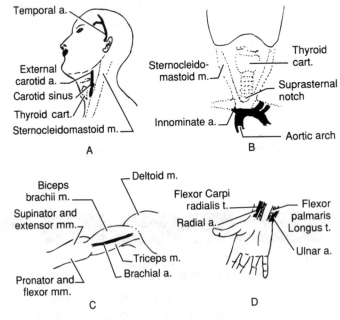

FIGURE 3-1 • Sites of palpable arteries.
(Reproduced with permission from LeBlond RF, *DeGowin RL, Brown DD: DeGowin's Diagnostic Examination*, 9th edition. New York, NY: McGraw-Hill; 2008. Figure 4-2.)

Leg

Femoral: Under the inguinal ligament in the groin area.

Popliteal: Deep in the soft area of the posterior knee.

Posterior tibial: Below the medial malleolus in the groove between the medial malleolus and the Achilles tendon.

Dorsalis pedis: Dorsum of the foot; below, proximal to and parallel to the great toe.

Heart

Apical: Between the fourth and fifth intercostal space, left side, midclavicular line in an adult.

Respirations

After the healthcare provider counts the pulse for 30 seconds, he/she will then count the patient's respirations for the next 30 seconds. The healthcare provider keeps his/her fingers on the patient's wrist so that the patient will be unaware of counting the respirations, and hence the respirations will not be altered. Respirations should normally be between 12 and 20 breaths per minute in the adult patient. The respiratory rate in an infant is faster than that in the adult, and is usually between 25 and 55 breaths per minute. The respiratory rate in a child can be from 14 to 40 breaths per minute depending on the child's age. The respiratory rate can change with exercise, anxiety, fever, and disease. The respiratory rate is counted by observing the rise and fall of the chest (see Table 3-3). One respiratory breath is equivalent to one inspiration

TABLE 3-3 Normal Respiratory Rate Levels		
Stage	**Age Range**	**Respiratory Rate, Breaths per Minute**
Newborn	Birth to 3 mo	35-55
Infant	3-6 mo	30-45
	6-12 mo	25-40
Toddler	1-3 y	20-30
Preschooler	3-6 y	20-25
School-aged child	6-12 y	14-22
Adolescent and adult	Over 12 y	12-20

(rise) and one expiration (fall) of the chest. The healthcare provider records the rate, rhythm, and depth of the patient's respirations. The patient's respirations should be relaxed, unlabored, without noise, and with equal and bilateral chest expansion.

Blood Pressure

It is important for the healthcare provider to assess the patient's blood pressure to evaluate the patient's cardiac output, blood volume, and elasticity of the arteries. The healthcare provider evaluates the systolic and diastolic blood pressure. The systolic blood pressure represents the left ventricle during contraction (systole) and the diastolic blood pressure represents the elastic recoil of the arteries or the resting state of the ventricles. A pulse pressure is the difference between the systolic blood pressure and the diastolic blood pressure, and represents the stroke volume: The amount of blood ejected from the heart with each beat. The pulse pressure increases with age due to the loss of elasticity (compliance) of the aorta. The patient's blood pressure can vary with: age, gender, race, ethnicity, obesity, anxiety, exercise, pain, fever, nicotine, caffeine intake, and medications. The blood pressure can also change with a patient's position. In the supine position, the blood pressure is the lowest because of decreased resistance; and it is the highest when the patient is standing, due to gravity. The blood pressure will vary during the day as the patient's activities change (see Table 3-4).

TABLE 3-4 Blood Pressure Stages		
Blood Pressure Stages		
Normal	120 mm Hg or less/ 80 mm Hg or less	Check yearly.
Hypotension	Less than 90 mm Hg/less than 60 mm Hg	Treat underlying condition.
Prehypertension	120-139/80-90 mm Hg	Check in 6 mo.
Stage 1 hypertension	140-159/90-99 mm Hg	Check within 2 mo.
Stage 2 hypertension	Greater than 160/ 100 mm Hg	Recheck in 1 wk or if greater than 180/100 mm Hg, treat immediately.

Technique

The healthcare provider measures the patient's blood pressure using a stethoscope and a sphygmomanometer. The patient is seated comfortably with their back supported, both feet on the floor, or in the supine or semi-Fowler position, and should be at rest for 5 minutes before taking the blood pressure. The arm should be supported at heart level to ensure an accurate reading. The patient's clothing on the arm should be removed. It is important to check that all equipment is in working order and has been calibrated. The healthcare provider needs to ensure use of a proper-sized blood pressure cuff according to the patient's arm and thigh sizes, available for infants, children, small adults, adults, and large adults. A cuff that is of incorrect size will result in a false reading. In the adult, 75% of the cuff should encircle the patient's arm, whereas in the child 100% of the cuff should encircle the arm. The patient's arm should be at the same level as the patient's heart. The healthcare provider palpates the brachial artery and places the cuff about 1 inch above the brachial artery. Most blood pressure cuffs have an arrow to line up the brachial artery with the blood pressure cuff. Encircle the cuff snugly around the patient's arm and place two fingers of your nondominant hand over the radial artery. Tighten the screw valve of the bulb and then inflate the cuff using the bulb with the dominant hand continuing to inflate the cuff about 30 mm Hg after which the radial pulse can no longer be palpated. This technique will estimate the systolic blood pressure and prevent missing an auscultatory gap; that is, no Korotkoff sounds (see Figure 3-2). The Korotkoff sounds are the arterial sounds heard through the stethoscope when taking a patient's blood pressure. Place the stethoscope (the bell or diaphragm are equally applicable) over the brachial artery, tighten the screw valve of the bulb, and inflate the cuff to the predetermined point (ie, 30 mm Hg above the loss of the radial pulse). Release the screw valve and deflate the cuff slowly, listening for the first sound (systolic blood pressure) and then continuing to listen until the last sound (diastolic blood pressure) is heard. After the last sound is heard, continue to deflate the cuff slowly for another 20 mm Hg and then, with the absence of sounds, deflate the cuff completely. The first and last sounds are recorded as the blood pressure (see Figure 3-2). The healthcare provider should wait a few minutes before attempting to take the blood pressure in the same arm to avoid venous congestion. A baseline blood pressure is recorded, however; hypertension is diagnosed after two to three abnormal readings. If the blood pressure is above 180/100 mm Hg, the patient should be referred immediately for treatment.

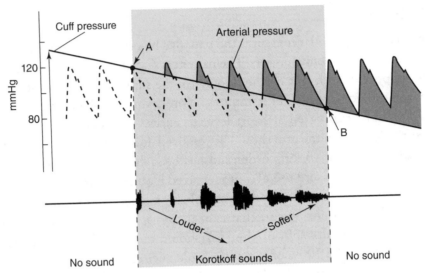

FIGURE 3-2 • Blood pressure measurement by auscultation. Point A indicates systolic blood pressure and point B indicates diastolic blood pressure.
(Reproduced with permission from Mohrman DE, *Heller LJ: Cardiovascular Physiology*, 7th edition. New York, NY: McGraw-Hill; 2011. Figure 6-9.)

Thigh Blood Pressure

Occasionally, the healthcare provider may need to take a patient's blood pressure using the upper leg to compare the arm pressure with the leg pressure. The leg pressure is normally higher than the arm pressure. Place the patient in the prone position and wrap a large blood pressure cuff around the lower third of the thigh. Place the stethoscope over the popliteal artery and take the patient's blood pressure using the same method employed for arm blood pressure. The leg reading is normally 10-40 mm Hg higher than that in the arm. An abnormal reading would reveal a lower leg blood pressure than the arm blood pressure.

ALERT

Orthostatic Changes in Blood Pressure
   Perform postural blood pressure to check for changes, if the healthcare provider suspects dehydration or if the patient complains of dizziness.

- Have the patient lie supine quietly for 2-3 minutes.
- Take the blood pressure and pulse in the supine position.
- Assist the patient to the sitting position and take the blood pressure and pulse again.

- Assist the patient to the standing position and take the blood pressure and pulse for the third time.
- Record the findings.

  An orthostatic change of systolic blood pressure greater than 20 mm Hg and a pulse increase of greater than 20 beats per minute is abnormal and can occur with increasing age, hypovolemia, and various medications.

Electronic Equipment

In many settings, the healthcare provider may use electronic equipment to take the patient's temperature, pulse, or blood pressure. It is important to remember that the equipment needs to be checked frequently to ensure that it is in good working order. The accuracy of the equipment is dependent on using the correct blood pressure cuff according to the size of the patient's arm or thigh. The equipment needs to be calibrated according to the manufacturer's instructions. If the healthcare provider obtains an abnormal reading, then the patient's blood pressure should be rechecked by the manual method. Electronic equipment should not be used if the patient is having tremors, seizures, or has an irregular heart rate.

REVIEW QUESTIONS

1. **The term prehypertension is defined as a blood pressure between which of the following ranges?**

   A. 90/60-110/60 mm Hg

   B. 120/80-139/90 mm Hg

   C. 150/90-160/100 mm Hg

   D. 160/100-180/100 mm Hg

2. **A patient's temperature can vary with which of the following factors?** *Select all that apply.*

   A. Stress

   B. Age

   C. Time of day

   D. Gender

   E. Eye color

3. The healthcare provider is preparing to take the patient's blood pressure and understands that the patient should initially:

   A. rest quietly for 5 minutes.
   B. drink 4 oz of water.
   C. elevate the legs.
   D. lie in the prone position.

4. The healthcare provider takes the adult patient's respiratory rate and counts 26 breaths in 1 minute. The healthcare provider would document this as:

   A. bradypnea.
   B. eupnea.
   C. tachypnea.
   D. dyspnea.

5. The healthcare provider takes the patient's blood pressure when the patient is lying, sitting, and then standing, and obtains a difference of 30 mm Hg from the lying position to standing position. The healthcare provider recognizes that this could be caused by:

   A. hypervolemia.
   B. asthma.
   C. decreased blood volume.
   D. ethnicity.

6. The arterial sounds the healthcare provider hears through the stethoscope when taking a patient's blood pressure are called?

   A. Normal sounds
   B. Korotkoff sounds
   C. Pulse sounds
   D. Carotid sounds

7. Which of the following is the least reliable method for taking a patient's temperature?

   A. Temporal
   B. Tympanic
   C. Oral
   D. Axillary

8. The amplitude of the normal pulse is:

   A. 1+
   B. 2+
   C. 3+
   D. 4+

9. **The patient should not be aware of the healthcare provider taking the respiratory rate to avoid:**
   A. increased anxiety of the patient.
   B. altering the rate of respirations.
   C. changing the pulse rate.
   D. bilateral chest expansion.

10. **The healthcare provider takes the pulse of a 5-year-old child and notes that the rhythm increases with inspiration and decreases with expiration. The healthcare provider documents this as:**
   A. bradycardia.
   B. tachycardia.
   C. pulse deficit.
   D. sinus arrhythmia.

ANSWERS

1. B. Prehypertension is defined as a blood pressure in the range of 120-139/ 80-90 mm Hg.

2. A, B, C, D. Affects the patient's core body temperature.

3. A. The patient should initially rest for 5 minutes before the healthcare provider takes the blood pressure.

4. C. Respirations greater than 20 breaths per minute in the adult are defined as tachypnea. Bradypnea is respirations less than 12 breaths per minute and eupnea is between 12 and 20 breaths per minute. Dyspnea is when the patient is having difficulty breathing.

5. C. Decreased blood volume or hypovolemia can cause a change in the blood pressure when the patient changes position from lying to sitting or standing.

6. B. Korotkoff sounds are the arterial sounds the healthcare provider hears through the stethoscope when taking a patient's blood pressure.

7. D. The axillary method is the least reliable method to take the patient's temperature. The other methods are more reliable if done correctly.

8. B. 2+ is the normal amplitude of the pulse. The abnormal pulse ranges are: 0 is no pulse; 1+ is a weak, thready pulse; and 3+ is a bounding pulse.

9. B. The healthcare provider should count the patient's respiratory rate without the patient's awareness to avoid altering the rate of respirations.

10. D. Sinus arrhythmia. Bradycardia is a pulse less than 60 beats per minute, tachycardia is a pulse greater than 100 beats per minute, and a pulse deficit is the difference between the radial and peripheral pulse.

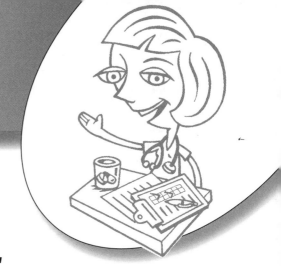

chapter 4

Assessment of Mental Status

LEARNING OBJECTIVES

After reviewing this chapter, the learner will be able to:

1 Discuss the appropriate information to gather during an interview.

2 Demonstrate an appropriate assessment of mental status.

3 List normal assessment findings.

4 Describe abnormal assessment findings.

5 Discuss the age-related differences related to mental status assessment.

> ## KEY WORDS
>
> | | |
> |---|---|
> | Clang associations | Perseveration |
> | Echolalia | Registration |
> | Flight of ideas | Schizophasia |
> | Intellectual functioning | Selective mutism |
> | Loose association | Thought content |

Introduction

A mental status examination is often conducted indirectly during the course of an interview and physical examination. The patient's verbal and nonverbal communication is constantly viewed and interpreted by many healthcare providers involved in their care. Evaluation of an individual's mental status during any single encounter reveals their current status at that point in time. Multiple assessments may be needed to determine the patient's overall mental status. Patients being seen by a neurologist or psychiatrist will have a more detailed evaluation of mental status. An initial evaluation is completed to determine a baseline and, periodically thereafter depending on the initial findings, specifics of expected disease progression, and any changes in status.

Assessment of mental status is important to identify memory loss, cognitive ability, disordered thought processes, or other alteration in mental status. Family members or caregivers may be the ones to initially identify that there has been a change in the patient's mental status.

Review of Anatomy and Physiology

The central nervous system receives information from neurons, processes, and then transmits it to the rest of the body. The individual cells responsible for the transmission of impulses are called neurons. The number of neurons that a patient has is fixed and the cells do not regenerate if damaged. Neurotransmitters are substances that help the information travel from one neuron to the next. Neurotransmitters within the brain are involved in a variety of functions (see Table 4-1).

Multiple neurotransmitters are involved in many of the body's day-to-day functions. Individual neurotransmitters may have levels above or below the

TABLE 4-1 Function of Neurotransmitters within the Brain									
	Mood	Movement	Learning	Memory	Sleep	Attention and Alertness	Appetite	Energy	Libido
Acetylcholine		X	X	X	X				X
Dopamine	X	X	X	X		X		X	X
Norepinephrine	X			X	X	X	X	X	X
Epinephrine					X	X		X	X
Serotonin	X				X	X	X		X
Glutamine		X	X	X				X	

normal level, which result in changes to mood, movement, learning, memory, sleep, attention, focus and alertness, appetite, energy, and libido (see Table 4-2).

Subjective Information

Interview

A single encounter may be insufficient to fully assess the patient's mental status. Some alterations in mental status are intermittent and may not be obvious during the first encounter. During any individual encounter, the patient may appear to have intact cognitive function or recall during the encounter and have episodes of impairment at other times. Early in the appearance of dementia (eg, Alzheimer disease), symptoms are often intermittent. Family members, who spend longer periods of time with the patient, can be helpful in identification of altered cognitive ability at other times. Remember to respect the patient's privacy. You should obtain the patient's consent to speak with family members whenever possible. Maintain patient privacy and basic comforts during the interview. Always introduce yourself to the patient before the interview or examination and tell the patient the purpose of the encounter.

Establishing a rapport with the patient allows for a more accurate evaluation of their mental status. Awareness of cultural differences in communication is also important in the interpretation of patient responses. In some cultures, it is believed that direct eye contact is an important component of nonverbal communication, signifying self-confidence and interest in what the other person is saying. In others, it is believed that sustained eye contact is inappropriate, especially between men and women. In yet other cultures, sustained eye contact

TABLE 4-2 Related Health Effect of Abnormal Neurotransmitter Levels

	Acetylcholine	Dopamine	Norepinephrine	Epinephrine	Serotonin	-Aminobutyric acid (GABA)	Glutamine
Anxiety		Increased	Increased	Increased	Decreased	Decreased	Decreased
Depression	Increased	Decreased	Decreased	Decreased	Decreased		Increased
Dementia	Decreased						
Psychosis		Increased					
Parkinson disease (movement and cognitive changes)		Decreased					Increased
Schizophrenia		Increased	Increased	Increased			Decreased
Attention disorders		Increased					Increased

may be interpreted as a challenge. It may be considered a sign of respect to divert direct eye contact in few other cultures. Likewise, awareness of normal age-related decline in hearing or vision must be taken into consideration.

Use of open-ended questions allows the patient to explain or elaborate their answers. Allow the patient time to answer the questions that you have asked without interrupting. Be aware of nonverbal communication during the interview, such as body position, movements, eye contact, volume, and tone of voice.

Review of Systems (ROS)

Alterations in mental status may result in other signs or symptoms that indicate something is amiss. Some patients will present with a physical complaint (insomnia, pain, etc) that is caused by alteration in mental status. In older patients, an altered mental status may be indicative of a physical condition. Some geriatric patients experiencing a significant infection (eg, urosepsis) will present with altered mental status rather than fever and urinary symptoms.

General: Fatigue and weight loss are nonspecific, common symptoms that can be due to a variety of causes, both physical and mental. Depression or dementia may result in alteration in nutrition and weight loss. A depressed patient may feel more fatigued.

HEENT: Headaches, visual changes, hearing changes, loss of smell, vertigo, dizziness, or loss of balance may be the result of pathology of the central nervous system.

Peripheral: Numbness, tingling, burning, or loss of sensation may occur as a result of peripheral neurologic damage due to disorders such as diabetes or multiple sclerosis. Patients with peripheral neurologic disorders may have coexisting central nervous system symptoms.

Pain: Ask the patient about the presence of pain. Depression is not uncommon in patients with chronic pain conditions, which may impact mental status function.

Risk Evaluation

A family history of certain mental health disorders increases the likelihood of the patient developing a similar disorder. For example, schizophrenia is more common in those patients with a family history of the disorder.

Eating disorders (such as anorexia nervosa or bulimia) are more common in adolescents and occur in both genders, but are more common in girls.

Substance use, such as cannabis, increases the risk of psychotic symptoms.

Patients with a history of uncontrolled hypertension, diabetes, or hyperlipidemia all have an increased risk of cerebrovascular accident. These coexisting morbidities increase the risk of developing a vascular dementia.

Objective Information

Equipment Needed

None.

Assessment Techniques

Inspection, interview.

Physical Examination

The mental status assessment should be conducted with a systematic approach and begins with the initial contact with the patient. Look at the patient's overall behavior and appearance. The condition of some patients (intoxicated, severe pain, altered levels of consciousness) will necessitate prioritizing the examination to get the essential information first. To help organize the mental status examination, you need to include assessment of the overall appearance, attitude, and affect (outward show of emotion); physical activity; mood (an underlying sustained emotion); speech; though content and process; higher level (intellectual) functioning; insight and judgment.

Overall Appearance, Attitude, and Affect

How is the patient's overall attitude or affect? The patient's attitude and affect should be appropriate to the situation. Is there a rapport with the interviewer or other personnel in the room? Is the patient dressed appropriately for the time of year and setting? Are they well groomed? A change or decline in cognitive function may present as a lack of attention to detail, resulting in inappropriate attire or obvious lack of grooming. The patient's facial expressions should be appropriate to the setting and match the words and inflection of their voice. Is the patient able to focus on the task at hand—the interview? Lack of attention span may be indicative of cognitive impairment or mental health disorders. The patient's affect is typically described as appropriate, constricted (a reduced range of emotion), flat (lacking emotion, appearing detached from the situation), labile, incongruent, hostile, or shallow.

Alertness

Is the patient awake and alert or is the level of consciousness compromised? Assessment of the patient's behavior and responsiveness can help in determining the level of consciousness.

An altered level of consciousness may be indicative of an underlying dysfunction of the brain or physiologic cause (lack of tissue oxygenation, altered blood sugar levels, intoxication, and effect of sedatives or analgesics).

The AVPU scale is a simple way to determine the level of consciousness. The abbreviation AVPU represents alert, response to verbal stimuli, response to painful stimuli, and unresponsiveness.

Begin by determining the level of alertness. Patients who are alert are aware of their surroundings and are able to interact. Patients who are less alert (sleepy, mildly sedated, intoxicated, or with neurologic disease) may respond to verbal stimulation, such as calling their name. In patients with no response to verbal stimuli, it is appropriate to check response for painful stimulation. Pinching the skin between the thumb and index finger or the lower portion of the nail may elicit a response. The patient may have a purposeful response to pain or a less specific response. Patients who do not respond are considered unresponsive.

ALERT

The range of a patient's level of consciousness can be any of the following:

- Conscious (alert and oriented)
- Confused (disoriented, difficulty following instructions)
- Delirious (disoriented, restless, agitated, altered attention)
- Somnolent (drowsy, mumbling responses)
- Obtunded (sleepy, slowed responses)
- Stuporous (minimal spontaneous activity, withdrawal response to painful stimuli, sleep-like)
- Comatose (not arousable, no response to painful stimuli, gag reflex, pupillary response)

Level of Orientation

Orientation is the awareness of current environment in relation to person, place, and time. In the setting of a head injury, you need to check if the patient is oriented to the event (injury) also. Does the patient recognize family members and friends? Do they know where they are? Can they correctly name the country, state, county, town, hospital, floor, room? Does the patient know their current age? Can the patient correctly name the season, the year, month, date, and day? Can they name the president? Disorientation to time usually occurs first, and may not be an indicator of mental health problems. Patients admitted to the hospital may experience difficulty in approximating the time of day, as their frame of reference has been altered.

Physical Activity

Does the patient appear at ease? Are they comfortable while stationary during the interview and examination? Do they appear calm, agitated, restless, or hypoactive? Excessive movement may be due to agitation, hyperactivity, or anxiety. Patients with limited motion and poor eye contact are in a different emotional state than the fidgety patient. Do you notice any abnormal movements (tics, unusual mannerisms, etc)? Are their movements coordinated?

Mood

The patient's mood is indicative of their sustained emotional state. Whereas affect can be fleeting, mood is more sustained. Does the patient appear relaxed or anxious; happy, angry, or sad; hopeful or hopeless; apathetic or euphoric? Are there any nonverbal cues to how the patient is feeling? Does the sad or depressed patient have any thoughts of suicide? If the patient does have any suicidal thoughts, ask if they have a plan. It is important to identify patients with suicidal ideation in order to intervene appropriately to keep the patient safe. You can also ask the patient if they have ever attempted suicide in the past, or had thoughts of hurting themselves or others. The mood is typically described as depressed, anxious, angry, euphoric (elated, excess happiness), or dysphoric (unhappy, ill at ease, distressed).

Speech

Listen to the choice of words, the volume, speed, and pattern of speech when the patient answers. Is the patient articulate? Is the speech spontaneous and conversational, at a comfortable volume, or is it unusually rapid or slow? Is the speech slurred, mumbled, stilted, or repetitive? If there are abnormalities in speech identified, are they new or normal for the patient? Is there normal inflection and tone of voice, or is it a monotone speech pattern?

Echolalia is a repetitive and uncontrollable repetition of words that have been spoken by someone else. This may be a normal developmental finding in young children as they mimic others.

Perseveration is an uncontrollable repetition of the same words over and over again. It may be seen in patients with traumatic brain injury, lesions within the frontal lobe, autism spectrum disorders, or in attention deficit hyperactivity disorder (ADHD).

Selective mutism occurs when a person who is capable of speech is unable to speak, typically in specific situations or to specific people. The patients converse normally in other settings. It may be seen with social anxiety disorder.

Clang associations or clanging describes a connection between words or ideas based on the sound. It may be seen in schizophrenia or in bipolar patients who are in a manic phase.

Thought Content and Process

Thought content refers to what the patient is thinking about and *thought process* refers to how the patient is thinking about those things. Are their thoughts relevant, logical, tangential, confusing, incoherent, or illogical?

Loose association refers to a disordered thought process where a series of ideas appear to lack a logical connection.

Flight of ideas is an almost continuous, rapid flow of speech that jumps from topic to topic and is seemingly unrelated, but may be prompted by word associations, environmental cues, etc. It can be disorganized and difficult to comprehend and is most commonly seen in schizophrenia or mania.

Word salad, or schizophasia, describes speech that is typical of a disordered thought process and is disorganized, lacking coherence and meaning and may contain neologisms (words that are created by the speaker). It is commonly seen in disoriented individuals (eg, dementia) and schizophrenia.

Delusions are an irrational, unshakable belief that something is true when it is not. The belief is held even when the patient is presented with information that disproves the belief. Delusions are not related to religious or cultural beliefs that may seem untrue to those outside the religion or culture. They can be categorized as grandiose (centered on the patient's own importance), persecutory (someone or something is out to get them), somatic (belief that something permanent is wrong with them, unlike hypochondriasis where the condition is temporary), jealousy, erotomanic (belief that someone else—possibly a celebrity—is in love with them), or mixed (combination of two or more of the above). Patients with dementia may experience delusions. Delusions may be accompanied by hallucinations or paranoia. Examples of some common delusions include grandeur, persecution, nihilism (the belief that nothing exists, seen in schizophrenia), somatic, or being under alien control. They may be seen in psychosis, schizophrenia, or bipolar disorder.

Hallucinations refer to the sensation of something that appears to be real and may include tactile (feeling of crawling on the skin), auditory (hearing sounds that are not there, such as music, doors closing), hearing voices (complimentary, critical, neutral, or offering commands) when no one is speaking, visual (seeing things that are not there, such as patterns, objects), and olfactory (smelling an odor that is not there). Hearing voices is the most common hallucination and may result in harm to the patient or others if the commands are followed. Patients who are intoxicated or coming off of substances (eg, Lysergic acid diethylamide [LSD], crack) may experience hallucinations. Patients with delirium, dementia, temporal lobe epilepsy, high fever, schizophrenia, psychosis, and sensory impairment may experience hallucinations.

Illusions are misleading or inappropriate perceptions of external stimuli. The stimulus is real and is not properly interpreted.

Paranoia refers to the perception of being personally threatened or feeling that someone or something is "out to get" or harm you. Patients experiencing paranoia may feel distrust and suspicious or appear hostile and imagine that others are talking about them behind their backs. In some instances, the patient may feel that others can read their mind or that they can control other people's thoughts or actions with their own thoughts. Paranoia is seen in schizophrenia and paranoid personality disorder. It may also occur with dementia, Huntington disease, Parkinson disease, or following cerebrovascular accidents. Alcohol and certain medications or drugs (amantadine, amphetamines, H2 blockers, marijuana, ecstasy, phencyclidine [PCP or angel dust], LSD) can also induce paranoia.

Cognitive and Higher Level Functioning

Registration is the ability to learn something new or record a new memory. To assess registration, name three objects (eg, tree, dog, and apple) and ask the patient to repeat them. Use random words (eg, house, sand, and elephant), not the items that you see in the room (table, clock, chair, etc) which may offer visual cues to the patient. Allow multiple attempts until all three items are correct.

Memory (remote, recent): Attention and concentration are needed for memory. Ask the patient verifiable information about a recent event (what they had for breakfast) and a remote memory (the address of the house they grew up in). Ask the patient to name a common object (eg, a pen or a watch). Assess recall ability by asking the patient to tell you the three words that you told them earlier.

Intellectual functioning includes general information (or fund of knowledge), calculation, the ability to abstract, and comprehension. Fund of knowledge describes the overall level of information mastery and breadth of knowledge. Ask about recent social or political events. The questions should take into account the patient's background and interest. Not all patients are interested in the latest entertainment industry gossip or the current political debate.

Have the patient follow a three-step command. Ask the patient to pick up a pen from the table, place the cap on it, and put it in the cup on the table.

Have the patient read and obey a simple written command, such as tap your right foot. Caution with non-English-speaking patients and those with poor literacy.

Ask the patient to write a sentence. Look for a subject, object, and verb. Ignore spelling errors.

Ask the patient to draw a familiar object, such as the face of a clock. Give a specific time (eg, 3:30) to depict on the face of the clock. Ask the patient to copy a geographic shape (intersecting hexagons or a three-dimensional cube). This allows assessment of visuospatial processing (Figure 4-1).

For *calculation*, have the patient perform serial sevens. Starting with 100 count backwards (subtract) 7 repeatedly (100, 93, 86, 79, 72, 65, 58, 51).

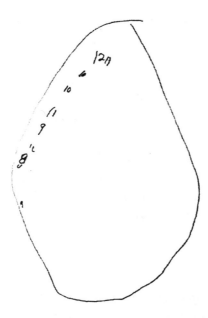

FIGURE 4-1 • Example of clock drawing for assessment of a patient's visuospatial processing. (Reproduced with permission from Ebert MH, Loosen PT, Nurcmbe B, Leckman JF: *Current Diagnosis & Treatment: Psychiatry*, 2nd edition. New York, NY: McGraw-Hill; 2008. Figure 6-6A.)

This can also be done with serial threes, subtracting 3 repeatedly (100, 97, 94, 91, 88, 85, 82, 79, 76, 73, 70). Always know the correct answers prior to asking questions such as these. For patient (or healthcare providers!) who have difficulty with mathematical calculation, ask the patient to spell a five-letter word backwards, such as "world" (D L R O W) or "beach" (H C A E B).

Abstract thought describes the ability to connect different things based on conceptual similarity. Ask the patient to interpret a common proverb, such as "people in glass houses shouldn't throw stones" or "you can't make an omelet without breaking a few eggs." The ability to think abstractly develops in adolescence.

Insight and Judgment

Insight is the ability to recognize that a problem exists and understand what options exist. Insight is necessary for the patient to comply with treatment recommendations and identify abnormal events (such as hallucinations). Judgment is a necessary component for problem solving.

Avoid the use of "why" questions as patients may not have the insight to be able to answer.

Expected Findings

The patient should be alert and oriented to time, place, and person. In the setting of a minor head injury (eg, softly bumping their head while getting out of their car), the patient should also be oriented to the event. Their mood should be appropriate to the setting. It is not unusual for a patient to be mildly anxious or uncertain of what to expect in a healthcare encounter. The patient should be appropriately groomed and dressed in a way that is seasonally appropriate. There will be variations in dress based on age, gender, culture, religious observation, etc. The patient should appear to be fairly comfortable with no unusual movements and their speech pattern should be spontaneous and conversational. The thought content and processes should be relevant and logical. Cognitive and higher level intellectual functioning should be intact.

Abnormal Findings

Disorientation is abnormal. The cause of disorientation needs to be established as it may be reversible in some cases, or indicative of a deterioration of a patient's condition in the setting of head injury. Altered mood may be indicative of mental health disorders or a result of physiologic changes. Differences in mood and affect are not typical. Lack of grooming may be due to situational conditions (being homeless) or due to altered mental status. Tics, constant fidgeting, or other movement (eg, pacing) may be indicative of either neurologic or mental status conditions. Altered speech patterns may indicate altered thought processes. Alteration in cognitive abilities may be due to neurologic disorders such as Alzheimer disease.

Hyperactivity, fidgeting, or twitching are considered abnormal findings. The cause of the excessive movements should be determined. Excessive, rapid, slurring, repetition, and minimal or excess volume of speech are all abnormal. It is important to determine if these changes in speech are new, temporary, or chronic.

Age-Related Changes

Pediatric

There are challenges in assessing mental status in young children. Determining the level of orientation is difficult as they cannot tell you the current date, time, or give a precise location. Ask the child's parent (or caregiver) if the child's mental status appears typical for them. Consider the age of the child—stranger anxiety is age appropriate in toddlers. Assessment of memory is best completed by asking young children about their favorite game or who they like to play with.

Young children are more concrete in thought. During adolescence they develop the ability to think abstractly.

School performance is an indicator of intellectual functioning in children. Regression in development, or loss of a previously acquired skill, may indicate a neurodegenerative disorder and needs further evaluation in children.

Onset of schizophrenia occurs typically during adolescence or young adulthood. Childhood schizophrenia may begin during school age and is rare.

Depression is more likely to occur in adolescent girls, but adolescent boys are more likely to have suicidal ideation.

Geriatric

As people age, they may need more time to process information and formulate answers. Memory, both recent and remote, should remain intact. When memory impairment does occur, it is more common for recent memory to be impaired as remote memories were formed a long time ago. Mild forgetfulness is not uncommon in the geriatric population. There is a difference in a patient who forgot where they left their car keys and a patient who forgot why car keys are used. Mild forgetfulness can happen at any age. Mild cognitive impairment is more pronounced than forgetting where you left your keys and can progress to dementia. Patients with mild cognitive impairment have difficulties with memory, are often aware of the memory changes, and usually have no problems with everyday activities.

Dementia is more common in elderly patients. Most causes of dementia are degenerative in nature and, therefore, permanent. The most common form of dementia is Alzheimer disease. Vascular dementia is due to repeated episodes of ischemia (multiple small strokes) within the brain. Multiple sclerosis, Huntington disease, and central nervous system infections may also result in irreversible damage to the brain and result in dementia. Traumatic brain injury, normal pressure hydrocephalus, low levels of vitamin B_{12}, brain tumors, infections (such as syphilis), or chronic alcohol abuse may all cause dementia that may be reversed if identified and treated early.

Cultural Considerations

The openness of discussing mental health varies from one culture to another. Certain groups still view certain disorders as something the patient should be able to "snap out of" or "get over." It is important to recognize one's own viewpoint when evaluating another person's reactions to illness.

CASE STUDY

Liz is a 72-year-old single woman brought in for evaluation by her niece. Liz has become forgetful and "inappropriate" at times, according to her niece. Liz was undressing while sitting in her seat on a recent trans-Atlantic plane trip to visit family. She became rather annoyed when her niece asked her what she was doing and explained that she wanted to go to sleep and was getting ready for bed.

REVIEW QUESTIONS

1. The healthcare provider is interviewing a patient who is speaking in an almost continuous, rapid flow of speech, jumping from topic to topic in a way that is seemingly unrelated. The term that best describes this is:

   A. flight of ideas.
   B. echolalia.
   C. word salad.
   D. clanging.

2. The healthcare provider is interviewing Liz who stops the conversation periodically, as if to listen to something else. On further questioning, the healthcare provider discovers that she is hearing voices. This is an example of:

   A. delusion.
   B. hallucination.
   C. paranoia.
   D. flight of ideas.

3. The ability to think in the abstract develops in:

   A. toddlers.
   B. school-age children.
   C. adolescents.
   D. college-age young adults.

4. "Serial sevens" are part of assessing higher cognitive function. Which of the following best describes "serial sevens"?

   A. Ask the patient to spell a five-letter word backwards.
   B. Ask the patient to subtract 7 repeatedly, starting with 100.
   C. Starting with 0 have the patient add 7 to the previous number repeatedly.
   D. Ask the patient to name seven common household objects

5. Testing registration as part of a mental status examination is best described as:

   A. naming three objects and asking the patient to repeat them.
   B. asking patients which high school they attended.
   C. asking the patient to supply demographic information and insurance cards.
   D. determining the accuracy of calculation ability.

6. The healthcare provider is interviewing Liz and understands that mild forgetfulness is:

   A. fairly common in a geriatric population.
   B. can happen at any age.
   C. does not typically progress to dementia.
   D. All of the above.

7. Most causes of dementia are:

   A. transient.
   B. permanent.
   C. due to a long-standing infection, such as untreated syphilis.
   D. due to inadequate nutritional intake.

8. **Peripheral neurologic symptoms may be the result of peripheral nerve damage and**

   A. are often associated with physiologic disease, such as diabetes or multiple sclerosis.
   B. have a family history of mental health disorders.
   C. have altered levels of neurotransmitters.
   D. have an increased risk of cerebrovascular accidents.

9. **Neurotransmitters within the brain are substances that:**

   A. control respiration and heart rate.
   B. cause fatigue.
   C. help neurologic impulses travel from one neuron to the next.
   D. control metabolism.

10. **An indicator of intellectual functioning in children is:**

   A. the ability to construct or draw a three-dimensional image.
   B. the ability to describe the message behind common proverbs.
   C. the ability to perform complex mathematical equations.
   D. academic performance.

ANSWERS

1. A. Flight of ideas is an almost continuous, rapid flow of speech that jumps from topic to topic and is seemingly unrelated.

2. B. Delusions are an irrational, unshakable belief that something is true. Hallucinations refer to the sensation of something that appears to be real and may include tactile, auditory, visual, or olfactory. Paranoia refers to the perception of being personally threatened. Flight of ideas is an almost continuous, rapid flow of speech that jumps from topic to topic and is seemingly unrelated, but may be prompted by word associations, environmental cues, etc.

3. C. The ability to think abstractly develops in adolescence.

4. B. Starting with 100 count backwards (subtract) 7 repeatedly to assess serial sevens.

5. A. Registration is assessed by naming three objects and asking the patient to repeat them.

6. D. Mild forgetfulness can happen at any age, is not uncommon in the elderly, and does not typically progress to dementia.

7. B. Most causes of dementia are degenerative and permanent.

8. A. Peripheral neurologic symptoms may be the result of peripheral nerve damage and are often associated with physiologic disease, such as diabetes or multiple sclerosis.

9. C. Neurotransmitters within the brain are substances that help neurologic impulses travel from one neuron to the next.

10. D. An indicator of intellectual functioning in children is academic performance.

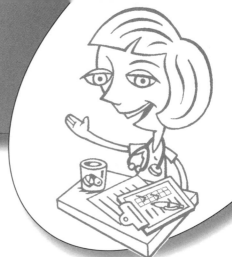

chapter 5

Assessment of the Skin, Hair, and Nails

LEARNING OBJECTIVES

After reviewing this chapter, the learner will be able to:

① Identify important anatomic landmarks of the skin.

② Discuss the appropriate information to gather during an interview.

③ Demonstrate a physical assessment of the skin.

④ List normal physical assessment findings.

⑤ Describe abnormal physical assessment findings.

⑥ Discuss the age-related differences related to the skin.

KEYWORDS

Alopecia

Basal cell carcinoma

Cyanosis

Erythema

Keloid

Macule

Melanoma

Nevus

Squamous cell carcinoma

Subcutaneous fat

Review of Anatomy and Physiology

The skin is considered the largest organ of the body and consists of three layers: epidermis (outer layer), dermis (middle layer), and the subcutaneous fat (inner layer) that connects the dermis to the underlying tissues (see Figure 5-1). The primary functions of the skin are to defend the body from foreign materials, especially microorganisms; help to regulate body heat; and retain moisture.

The epidermis layer covers the outermost areas of the body and consists of the keratinocyte cells that produce a fibrous protein called keratin that protects the skin and along with elastin and collagen strengthens the skin. Melanocytes are the pigment-producing cells located at or in the basal layer of the epidermis. The number of melanocytes present is consistent in everyone, but it is the proportions of melanin produced that determines the skin color along with other factors, such as exposure to sun, genetics, carotene pigment, and the underlying vascular bed.

The dermis separates the outer epidermis from the subcutaneous fat layer. The dermis layer nourishes the epidermis by papillae from the dermis that project into the epidermal region. Capillaries in the papillae diffuse nutrients into the epidermis. Structures found in the dermis are the blood vessels, nerves, lymphatic vessels, hair follicles, and the sebaceous glands that produce sebum to lubricate the skin and prevent fluid loss. The sweat glands, apocrine and eccrine, are found in the dermis and are important in the regulation of body temperature.

The subcutaneous layer consists of connective tissue and adipose tissue that supports the outer layers of the skin. This layer provides insulation for heat regulation.

Hair and nails are considered appendages of the skin. Hair originates from the hair follicles in the dermis. Adults have two types of hair: vellus and terminal. Vellus is hypopigmented and located all over the body, whereas terminal hair is found on the scalp, eyebrows, and eyelids. On puberty, terminal hair

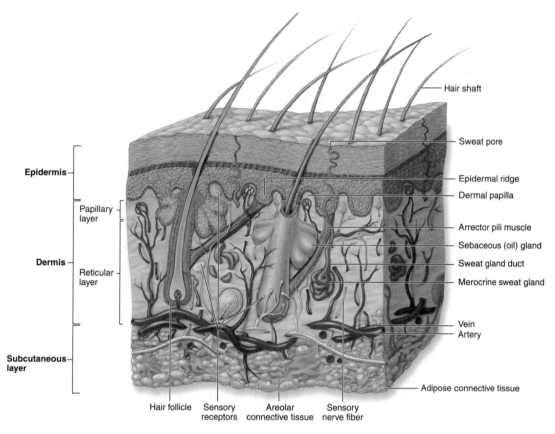

FIGURE 5-1 • An illustration of the skin anatomy.
(Reproduced with permission from Mescher AL: *Junqueira's Basic Histology: Text & Atlas*, 12th edition. New York, NY: McGraw-Hill; 2010. Figure 18-1.)

develops on the legs, axillae, and suprapubic areas, as well as the face, chest, or back of males. The color of terminal hair depends on pigment production. Hair serves to protect the body and filter dust and other debris. Nails are composed of hardened keratin plates and are found on the ends of the fingers and toes (see Figure 5-2). The nail plate is translucent and provides information about the oxygenation of the tissue below.

Subjective Information

Interview

Review of Systems

Ask the patient the following specific questions related to the skin assessment:
Are you experiencing any recent changes in your skin, which include dryness,

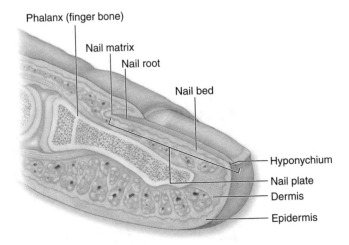

FIGURE 5-2 • An illustration of the nail anatomy.
(Reproduced with permission from Mescher AL: *Junqueira's Basic Histology: Text & Atlas*, 12th edition. New York, NY: McGraw-Hill; 2010. Figure 18-14.)

moisture, itching, rashes, lesions, color, odor, amount of perspiration, pain, numbness, swelling, or changes in mole or warts. Do you have any current problems with hair loss, changes in texture, color, or distribution? Have you noticed any changes in your nails, which include changes in color, separation from the nail bed, and brittleness? If the patient experiences any changes in the skin, it is important to determine the skin allergies or sensitivities that the patient experiences and treatments that have been effective.

Risk Factors Related to the System

Skin cancer is a form of cancer that develops in the tissues of the skin. There are three main types of skin cancer: Melanoma that develops in the melanocytes; basal cell cancer that develops in the lower part of the epidermis; and squamous cell cancer that develops in the squamous cells that form the surface of the skin. The risk factors for skin cancer include: exposure to ultraviolet radiation in the form of sunlight, tanning beds, and sunlamps. Other risk factors include: light skin and hair, a history of sunburns early in life, family history of skin cancer, and a personal history of skin cancer. Caucasians have the highest incidence rates of melanoma, Hispanic and American Indian/Alaska natives have the second highest, and Asian-Pacific Islanders and African Americans have the third highest. Latest statistics reveal that incidence and mortality rates are increasing among Caucasians.

Risk Evaluation

Patients at a higher risk of skin cancer have had one or more severe sunburns with blistering in childhood. The healthcare provider should ask the patient: Have you had any severe sunburn during childhood or recently? As the changes in nevi (moles) could indicate skin cancer, ask the patient: Have you noticed any recent changes in moles or birthmarks? To assess the risk of a skin infection, ask the patient if they have had any recent body tattoos or piercings. The patient who bites or picks his nails is at risk for nail infections: for example, paronychia—a local infection around the nail often at the cuticle with redness and swelling. Patients who braid their hair tightly or have frequent straightening or hair treatments are at risk for alopecia (loss of hair). The healthcare provider should ask the patient: Have you noticed any changes in hair after the treatment? Patients who use chemicals while working or while engaging in a hobby could have skin burns from the offending substance. Hence, ask the patient: Do you have exposure to environmental chemicals, dyes, or irritants in your employment or hobbies?

Self-Care Behaviors

Patients should wash their skin and hair with a mild soap and shampoo. Nails should be cleaned with a nail brush and dried thoroughly. Specific questions related to skin, nails, and hair care can alert patients at risk for xerosis (dry skin), infections of the nails, or hair loss. Ask the client about the use of sunscreen to assess the risk of skin cancers. The patient who frequents tanning salons is at a higher risk for skin cancers.

Objective Information

Equipment needed: Adequate direct lighting, gloves, small centimeter ruler, magnifying glass, and a Wood's light (to detect fungal infections of the skin). **Assessment techniques**: Inspection and palpation.

Physical Examination

Inspection

Inspection of the skin is the primary step in assessment of all body systems. Inspection of the skin is an important part of the assessment and should not be done with just a quick glance but should take a considerable amount of time. Start with the inspection of the hair on the head and work in a head-to-toe fashion, exposing only the area that is being examined. Move the limbs to look at the medial and posterior aspect of the arms and legs, and move the skin folds, for example, the area under the breasts. Intertriginous areas are located where the skin folds and the two areas rub together. Skin folds are commonly the warm and moist areas and are common spots for irritation and infection. Inspect each area of the body for color changes, intactness, lesions or rashes, and vascular changes of the skin.

Inspection of the hair starts with the inspection of the scalp, by separating the hair to reveal the skin underlying the hair. Note the color, consistency, and cleanliness of the hair. Inspection of the hair is performed at the same time as inspection of the skin, in a head-to-toe fashion.

Inspection of the nails starts when the healthcare provider shakes the patient's hand. Inspect the color of the fingernails and the underlying nail bed. Inspect the shape of the nails and note any markings.

Palpation

Palpation of the skin reveals temperature, moisture, texture, and thickness, swelling due to fluid in the underlying tissues (edema), mobility and turgor of the skin. Palpation is commonly performed without gloves avoiding areas where exudate or oozing from a lesion is present. Always use discretion when deciding to use gloves and don gloves when a lesion appears suspicious or contagious. Palpate the skin using the dorsum (back) of the hand to assess temperature and moisture of the skin. Using the fingertips assess the texture and thickness of the skin. Press the thumb or forefinger into the skin over a bony prominence at the ankle to determine the underlying fluid in the tissues. Gently pinch the skin between your thumb and forefinger under the clavicle to assess mobility and turgor of the skin.

Palpation of the scalp is performed after donning gloves and is performed concurrently with inspection.

Palpation of the nails reveals the surface texture. Assess the capillary refill by pinching one of the finger nails and the great toe and note the return of the color from pale to pink. Pink tone of the nail should return in 2-3 seconds. If the hands are cold to the touch, warm the hands first to prevent an abnormal positive finding.

Expected Findings

Inspection of the skin reveals an even pigmentation with hypopigmented areas on the palms of the hands and soles of the feet. Areas of sun exposure might reveal darker pigmented skin. Lesions or rashes are normally not present. Skin is intact without fissures (cracks), lesions, open wounds or lacerations, or uneven pigmentation.

Inspection of the hair reveals a color consistency without patches of hair loss. Inspection of the hair on the body should reveal vellus hair with coarse hair on the eyebrows and eyelashes. Hair distribution in the adult (after puberty) reveals hair in the axillae, groin, and legs. Male pattern of hair includes distribution of hair on the face and sometimes various degrees of hair on the chest, back, and arms.

Inspection of the nails reveals a round contour with a transparent nail and underlying pink tones. The skin at the base of the nails in not inflamed and is firmly attached to the base of the fingernail or toenail. There are no markings on the nail. The shape of the nail reveals a 160 degree angle between the base of the nail and the skin.

Palpation of the skin reveals the skin to be warm and dry bilaterally (comparing both sides of the body) with increased moisture in the axillae, groin, and intertriginous areas. Skin is thin with areas of thickness on the soles of the feet and palmar surfaces of the hands. The skin should feel soft and smooth to the touch. Edema should not be present and pinching of the skin should return it to its original position immediately.

Palpation of the nails reveals a smooth, firm surface. The nail bed should be firmly attached to the nail bed. Capillary refill should be under 2-3 seconds.

Palpation of the hair and scalp reveals hair that covers the entire scalp that is soft to the touch. No tumors or lesions are palpated on the scalp.

Abnormal Findings

The following skin color changes might be observed:

1. **Pallor**: Loss of color due to arterial insufficiency, anemia, or decreased oxygenation of the skin.
2. **Cyanosis**: Blue tinged, dull color due to loss of oxygenation of underlying tissues.
3. **Erythema**: Increase in red tones due to increased blood supply in the superficial capillaries seen with inflammation, fever, and blushing (see Figure 5-3).
4. **Jaundice**: Yellow skin tones due to increased amounts of bilirubin in the blood.

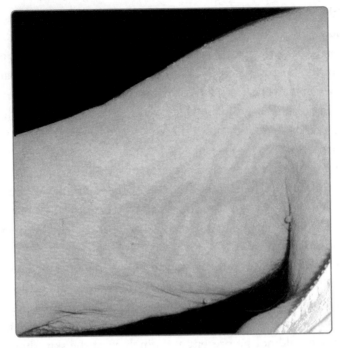

FIGURE 5-3 • An erythema.
(Reproduced with permission from Goldsmith LA, Katz SI, Gilchrest BA, et al: *Fitzpatrick's Dermatology in General Medicine*, 8th edition. New York, NY: McGraw-Hill; 2012. Figure 153-8.)

ALERT

If a lesion is found, the following should be documented:

1. Size in centimeters
2. Color distribution
3. Elevation
4. Configuration
5. Site on the body
6. Dry or oozing a substance

Common Primary Skin Lesions

Macule: A flat, brown, purple, or red lesion, which is less than 1 cm in width. For example, nevus (see Figure 5-4).

Patch: A flat, brown, purple, or red lesion, which is greater than 1 cm in width. For example, Mongolian spot.

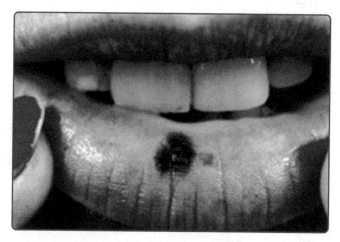

FIGURE 5-4 • A macule.
(Reproduced with permission from Goldsmith LA, Katz SI, Gilchrest BA, et al: *Fitzpatrick's Dermatology in General Medicine*, 8th edition. New York, NY: McGraw-Hill; 2012. Figure 5-9.)

Papule: A raised, solid lesion, less than 0.5 cm in width. For example, elevated nevus.

Plaque: Lesion formed of combined papules, which is larger than 1 cm in width. For example, psoriasis.

Nodule: A solid, elevated lesion, which can be firm or soft and less than 1-2 cm in width. For example, fibroma.

Tumor: A nodule greater than 2 cm in width. For example, carcinoma of the skin.

Vesicle: An elevated and fluid-filled lesion, which is less than 0.5 cm in width. For example, contact dermatitis.

Bulla: A vesicle larger than 0.5 cm in width. For example, burn blister.

Pustule: A pus-filled vesicle. For example, acne (see Figure 5-5).

Cyst: An encapsulated fluid-filled sac. For example, sebaceous cyst.

Wheal: An elevated, erythematous mass with irregular borders. For example, insect bite.

Common Secondary Skin Lesions

Fissure: A linear crack that may extend to the dermis of the skin.

Erosion: A loss of superficial epidermis that has a moist surface.

Excoriation: A superficial abrasion of the epidermis.

Ulcer: A deeper depression into dermis than erosion, which is irregular in shape and scars upon healing.

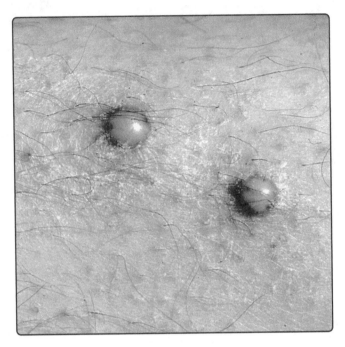

FIGURE 5-5 • A pustule.
(Reproduced with permission from Goldsmith LA, Katz SI, Gilchrest BA, et al: *Fitzpatrick's Dermatology in General Medicine*, 8th edition. New York, NY: McGraw-Hill; 2012. Figure 5-15.)

Scar: A healed tissue that is replaced with connective tissue and can appear as reddened initially and later as a lightened area in light-skinned patients and an area of darkened pigmentation in dark-skinned patients.

Keloid: A type of scarring where there is excessive collagen formation that appears raised and reddened in light-skinned patients and raised and hyper-pigmented in dark-skinned patients (see Figure 5-6).

Atrophy: Thinning of skin surface leaves markings that appear translucent.

Crust: A thick, dried exudate that varies in color from red to brown, black, or tan.

Scale: Shedding of dead keratin cells that appear dry and are white or silver in color.

Lichenification: Thickening of skin that is a result of scratching the skin.

Vascular Skin Lesions

Petechiae: A small, 1-3 mm red or purple macule caused by bleeding into the tissues.

Purpura: A patch of petechiae, usually greater than 3 mm in width.

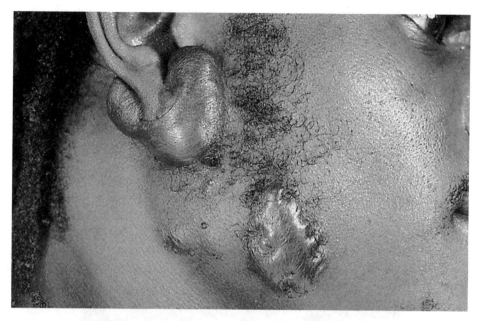

FIGURE 5-6 • A keloid.
(Reproduced with permission from Wolff K, Johnson RA: *Fitzpatrick's Color Atlas and Synopsis of Clinical Dermatology*, 6th edition. New York, NY: McGraw-Hill; 2009. Figure 9-51.)

Ecchymosis: Irregular macular lesions that result from bleeding into the tissues and appear red to black in color. On healing, the lesion changes to yellow and green.

Hematoma: An elevated ecchymosis.

Telangiectasias: Red lines, commonly in a spider-like shape, caused by dilated blood vessels.

Abnormal Nail Changes

Paronychia: A painful, red inflammation between the nail fold and nail plate, usually caused by bacteria or fungus.

Leukonychia: White spots on the nail resulting from trauma to the nail plate.

Onycholysis: The nail separates from nail bed and appears discolored (yellow, green, black) if a fungal infection is present or can result from nail trauma and appears white. It begins distally and progresses proximally.

Clubbing: The proximal edge of the nail elevated to greater than 180 degrees associated with long-standing oxygen deprivation to the periphery.

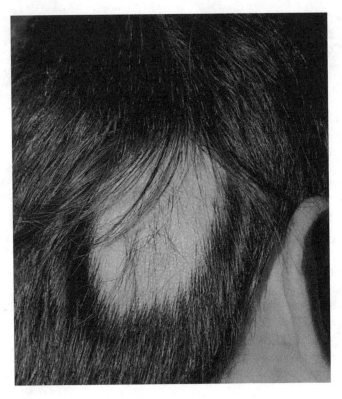

FIGURE 5-7 • Alopecia.
(Reproduced with permission from Wolff K, Johnson RA: *Fitzpatrick's Color Atlas and Synopsis of Clinical Dermatology*, 6th edition. New York, NY: McGraw-Hill; 2009. Figure 32-8.)

Koilonychia: A central depression of the nail, which is associated with iron deficiency.

Beau lines: Transverse depression of nail plate associated with trauma or disease.

Abnormal Hair Changes

Alopecia: Patchy hair loss resulting from trauma, illness, chemotherapy, or can be idiopathic (see Figure 5-7).

Folliculitis: Superficial infection of hair follicles that appears as pustules, with surrounding erythema.

Head lice: Nits in the hair that are best observed in the occipital area, which are small and translucent.

Tinea capitis: Patchy hair loss associated with a fungal infection of the scalp.

Hirsutism: Excessive body hair in females on the face, chest, arms, and legs, associated with endocrine abnormalities.

ALERT

Inspection of nevus (mole or freckle). If a nevus is found, the following may be used to evaluate the changes:

A = asymmetry: Is the nevus uniform on all sides?

B = border irregularity: Does the nevus have even borders, and if cut out could it be evenly folded?

C = color variation: Is the nevus all the same in color or does it vary in color??

D = diameter: How large is the nevus? Is it larger than 6 mm?

E = elevation: Is the nevus elevated?

F = frequency: Are there more than one nevus?

G = growing: Is the nevus growing or changing in size and shape?

**Cancer alert: Nevi that are asymmetrical, have irregular borders, changes in color, are greater than 6 mm, are elevated, or increasing in size are suspicious and needs to be evaluated by a healthcare practitioner specialized in dermatology.

If any of the above questions were answered affirmatively, then an urgent referral to a dermatologist should be made immediately.

Skin Cancer Examples

Basal cell carcinoma (BCC) is the most common type of skin cancer and is evidenced by a small papule that starts as colored skin or can be deeply pigmented (see Figure 5-8). It is translucent and shiny with telangiectasias (blood vessels in a spider-like pattern). The borders are rounded and pearly with a central depression. Basal cell cancer commonly grows slowly over several months or years and rarely metastasizes (spreads).

Squamous cell carcinoma (SCC) is the second most common type of skin cancer and is evidenced by a reddened scaly patch with sharp margins (see Figure 5-9). The center is ulcerated and the surrounding area has erythema (redness). It grows faster than BCC, but can be relatively slow in growth and rarely metastasizes.

Malignant melanoma is a form of skin cancer that starts in the pigment-producing cells called melanocytes. It is evidenced by a mole that has changed (see ABCDEFG above in Alert). Melanomas commonly develop on areas that are exposed to the sun, but can develop on unexposed areas also. The first sign

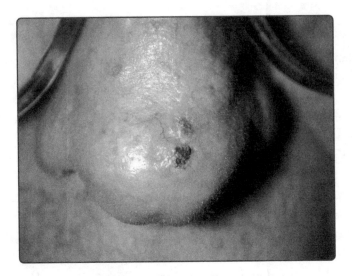

FIGURE 5-8 • A nodular type of BCC.
(Reproduced with permission from Goldsmith LA, Katz SI, Gilchrest BA, et al: *Fitzpatrick's Dermatology in General Medicine*, 8th edition. New York, NY: McGraw-Hill; 2012. Figure 115-1.)

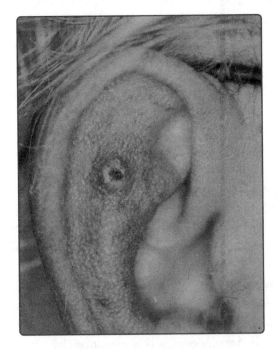

FIGURE 5-9 • A papular SCC of the ear.
(Reproduced with permission from Goldsmith LA, Katz SI, Gilchrest BA, et al: *Fitzpatrick's Dermatology in General Medicine*, 8th edition. New York, NY: McGraw-Hill; 2012. Figure 114-1.)

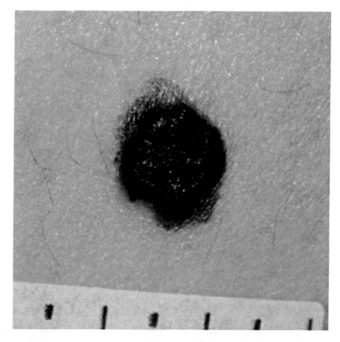

FIGURE 5-10 • Melanoma.
(Reproduced with permission from Wolff K, Johnson RA: *Fitzpatrick's Color Atlas and Synopsis of Clinical Dermatology*, 6th edition. New York, NY: McGraw-Hill; 2009. Figure 12-12.)

of a melanoma is a changed mole or nevus. Prognosis for this type of skin cancer depends on the depth and ulceration of the lesion when it is diagnosed. It commonly metastasizes to other areas of the body (Figure 5-10).

Age-Related Changes

Pediatric

Infants can have several variations in skin color. The skin and sclera of the eyes can appear yellow due to bilirubin in the blood and an immature liver. A dense collection of melanocytes can cause darkened areas of the infant's skin ranging in color from brown to blue-black in color and can resemble a bruise. They are more commonly called Mongolian spots and are found in children of African, Native American, Asian, and Hispanic descent. Flat, solitary macules ranging in color from light to dark brown can occur in infants and children of African and Hispanic descent in infancy and in Caucasians in childhood. These spots are commonly benign but should be investigated if found to be larger than 2-3 cm. Hemangiomas are common at birth and are due to an abnormal buildup of blood vessels in the skin. They appear as a red or red-purple raised lesion on the skin and are commonly found on the face and neck.

At puberty, sebaceous gland activity with resultant increase in sebum production, increase in androgens and bacteria on the skin produce acne. Papules, pustules, open comedones, and closed comedones usually appear on the face, chest, and back. Severe cases of acne can appear as a cyst that is an encapsulated fluid-filled mass. Cysts are commonly nodular and a referral to a dermatologist is needed for treatment. Acne usually decreases by 19 years of age, but can continue throughout adulthood (Figure 5-11). The apocrine glands mature in adolescence and produce an increase in sweat in the axillae and groin areas. The mixture of sweat and bacteria cause a foul-smelling odor.

Hair can become weak and break easily with poor nutrition. Severe protein deficiency in children can result in changes in the hair (pigmented areas) and skin (dry, flaky).

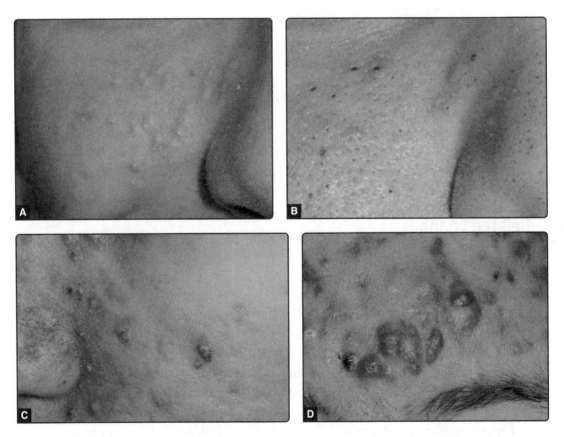

FIGURE 5-11 • Acne lesions. (A) Closed comedone. (B) Open comedone. (C) Inflammatory papule. (D) Nodule. (Reproduced with permission from Goldsmith LA, Katz SI, Gilchrest BA, et al: *Fitzpatrick's Dermatology in General Medicine*, 8th edition. New York, NY: McGraw-Hill; 2012. Figure 80-3.)

Geriatric

Skin changes in the older adults are commonly related to the amount of sun exposure over their lifetime. Senile lentigines are flat, brown, round areas on the skin, commonly called age spots or liver spots, and are not related to liver functioning though. Senile lentigines are found on sun-exposed areas and can be minimized with reducing sun exposure and wearing sunscreens. Seborrheic keratosis are raised, brown areas on the skin that look scaly or "pasted on" the skin. They are not precancerous. Actinic keratosis are yellow or pale raised areas that feel coarse (see Figure 5-12). They appear on sun-exposed areas and are considered to be precancerous. A cherry angioma is another normal variation that is typically not clinically significant. It appears as a round papule that is red or purple in color, usually seen on the torso and extremities. Observe all aging variations for changes in size, elevation, color, or distribution.

The skin in the older adult could be dry due to a decline in functioning of sweat and sebaceous glands. The skin is less elastic and skin does not return to its original position after being pinched, and hence decreasing the mobility of the skin. The skin splits easily causing an increased risk of infection because the skin is no longer intact.

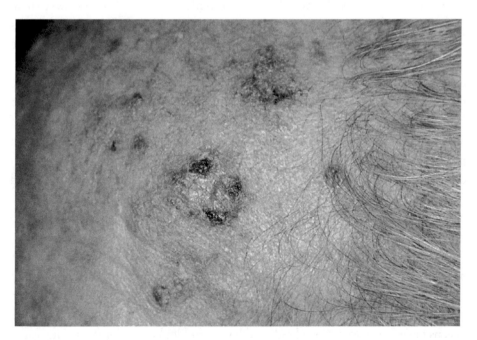

FIGURE 5-12 • Actinic keratosis.
(Reproduced with permission from Wolff K, Johnson RA: *Fitzpatrick's Color Atlas and Synopsis of Clinical Dermatology*, 6th edition. New York, NY: McGraw-Hill; 2009. Figure 10-26.)

The hair of the older adult gradually becomes gray due to a decreasing amount of functioning melanocytes. Male pattern balding is hereditary and starts with a receding hairline on either side of the forehead and progresses to the middle of the head. Hair is thinner in the older adult due to the decreasing function of the hair follicles. Women can develop hair on the chin or upper lip after menopause due to decreasing amounts of estrogen that leaves androgens unhindered.

The nails of the older adult can become thin and brittle and growth rates decline. The toenails become thick and can appear yellow. Peripheral vascular disease in the older adult can increase the risk of the individual having thick toenails.

Cultural Considerations

The patients with the highest risk of skin cancer are Caucasians; however, it is prudent for all patients to wear sunscreen. Melanin protects the skin from ultraviolet rays in darkly pigmented patients; however, the risk for dark-skinned patients is not zero. Mortality rates are high because an individual with dark skin is often diagnosed later than an individual with lighter skin. African Americans can develop melanomas in areas that are not pigmented, such as the soles of the feet, palms of the hands, and beneath the nails. Keloids are irregularly shaped scars formed after injury to the skin, which develop from excessive collagen production. It is a condition that is probably hereditary due to the fact that it is common in certain families. The scar is not cancerous but can cause cosmetic problems for the patient. After inflammation, the skin of a darker individual can become hypopigmented or hyperpigmented. Woman patients of African, Hispanic, Asian, Indian, and Mediterranean descent can develop hyperpigmented patches on the face with sun exposure called melasma. It commonly occurs in pregnancy (chloasma) or with certain medications (hormones) or cosmetics. Daily use of sunscreen is suggested to help prevent this condition.

The hair of individuals differs generally with variations in dryness, texture, and color. Cosmetic products can injure hair follicles and individuals who use extensive cosmetic products may complain of areas of hair loss (alopecia). An odor results when aprocrine gland secretions of sweat get mixed with bacteria. Asians have fewer aprocrine glands and have a milder body odor than Caucasians and individuals of African descent who have a stronger body odor than other ethnic groups.

CASE STUDY

Miss M is a 22-year-old Caucasian female who complains of several moles on her face, chest, and arms. The healthcare provider is interviewing the patient who stated "I go to the tanning salon three times a week because it is safer than sitting in the sun." Miss M has a history of ear infections as a child, and currently is not taking any medications. Medical history reveals that her father had a "suspicious lesion" removed from his left ear 2 years ago, but the patient is not aware of the diagnosis of the lesion. Her mother is alive and well. Miss M has two siblings, a brother and a sister, who have no prior history of skin disease. The patient is a nonsmoker, but admits to drinking three to four alcoholic beverages on the weekend. Miss M is requesting information on skin cancer prevention because her father had a suspicious lesion removed two years ago.

REVIEW QUESTIONS

1. **A patient with the greatest risk for skin cancer is:**
   A. a 35-year-old Hispanic female with a history of sunburns in childhood.
   B. a 45-year-old African American male with no previous history of cancer.
   C. a 30-year-old Asian-Pacific Islander male with a complaint of dry, itchy skin.
   D. a 25-year-old Caucasian female with no prior history of skin cancer.

2. **What determines the color of the skin?**
   A. The number of melanocytes.
   B. The amount of sebum produced.
   C. Exposure to ultraviolet light.
   D. Amount of melanin produced.

3. **Which of the following is the best response to Miss M's statement "I go to the tanning salon three times a week because it is safer than sitting in the sun."**
   A. "Tanning salons have less ultraviolet radiation than sitting in the sun."
   B. "Tanning salons are not safer than sitting in the sun."
   C. "Tanning salons can be safe if one wears sunscreen while tanning."
   D. "People with light skin should never go out in the sun!"

4. Basal cell carcinoma (BCC) originates in which part of the skin?

   A. Dermis
   B. Epidermis
   C. Aprocrine glands
   D. Subcutaneous layer

5. When performing the health history on Miss M, the healthcare provider understands that the most important question to ask about the moles on her face, chest, and arms is:

   A. Do you wear sunscreen in the summer?
   B. Do your siblings have similar moles on their face, chest, and arms?
   C. Have any of the moles changed in the past 6 months?
   D. How old was your father when the "suspicious lesion" on his skin was found?

6. The healthcare provider is evaluating Miss M's skin on her back and notes a lesion that has dry exudate. What should be done next?

   A. Call the physician immediately.
   B. Don gloves and continues to examine the lesion.
   C. Avoid the lesion and continue the examination.
   D. Call another person to come and examine the lesion with them.

7. The healthcare provider is examining Miss M's face and finds a nevus that is 2 × 3 cm flat and brown in color. The correct documentation is:

   A. a macule.
   B. a papule.
   C. a patch.
   D. a nodule.

8. Miss M states that her grandmother has a lesion on her face that is 1 × 2 cm, brown, raised, scaly, and looks "pasted" on her skin. This is most likely a:

   A. seborrheic keratosis.
   B. actinic keratosis.
   C. basal cell carcinoma (BCC).
   D. precancerous lesion.

9. Miss M stated that she is worried about losing her hair at an early age because her mother is starting to lose her hair. Hair loss (alopecia) in women can be caused by:

   A. use of cosmetic products.
   B. thyroid disease.
   C. vitamin deficiencies.
   D. all of the above.

10. **Miss M complains of "acne" on her chin and nose. Acne is commonly documented in the medical record as:**

    A. macules.

    B. pustules.

    C. wheals.

    D. plaque.

ANSWERS

1. A. A 35-year-old Hispanic female, who has a history of sunburns in childhood, is at the` highest risk for skin cancer. B and C are at a lower risk, and D although has light skin has no prior history of skin cancer and has a lower risk than A.

2. D. The color of the skin is determined by the amount of melanin produced by the melanocytes, and not by the number of melanocytes.

3. B. Miss M should be taught that tanning salons are not safer than sitting in the sunlight and that sunscreen does not protect one 100% from skin cancer. Miss M has light skin, especially with a family history of a "suspicious lesion," and is at a high risk for skin cancer.

4. B. Basal cell carcinoma (BCC) originates in the deepest layer of the epidermis (top layer of the skin).

5. C. If a mole (nevus) is changing, then it is suspicious and should be evaluated immediately by a healthcare practitioner specialized in dermatology.

6. B. The healthcare provider should don gloves before examining a lesion with any exudate or fluid oozing from it.

7. C. A patch is a macule that is larger than 1 cm, which is flat and not raised.

8. A. Seborrheic keratosis is usually brown, evenly colored, scaly, and raised, and looks pasted on the skin. It is not a precancerous lesion and is usually found on sun-exposed areas of the body.

9. D. Hair loss can result due to several different causes including: thyroid disease; vitamin deficiencies; zinc and other diet deficiencies; protein and fatty acids; and use of cosmetic products and procedures, braiding, and straightening.

10. B. Macules are flat and brown in color and are less than 1 cm in width; for example, nevus. Wheals are elevated lesions with irregular borders and are reddened; for example, insect bite. Plaque is formed by several papules combined together and is greater than 1 cm in width; for example, psoriasis.

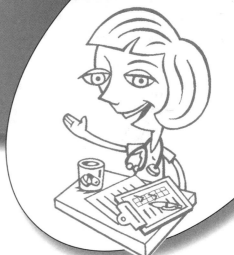

chapter **6**

Assessment of the Head, Eyes, Ears, Nose, and Throat (HEENT)

LEARNING OBJECTIVES

After reviewing this chapter, the learner will be able to:

1 Identify important anatomic landmarks of the head and neck.

2 Discuss the appropriate information to gather during an interview.

3 Demonstrate a physical assessment of the head and neck.

4 List normal physical assessment findings.

5 Describe abnormal physical assessment findings.

6 Discuss the age-related differences related to the head and neck.

KEYWORDS

Auricle
Fissure
Helix
Medial canthus
Nasal mucosa

Orbit
Oropharynx
Parotid glands
Sclera
Thyroid gland

Introduction

Much of the sensory information that reaches the brain is transmitted from the head and neck area. The senses of vision and hearing can help us to safely assess and interact with our environment. Taste impacts our food preferences and may affect our nutritional status. Speech allows us to communicate effectively with others.

Review of Anatomy and Physiology

In order to properly assess the head and neck area, an understanding of the normal anatomy and physiology is necessary. Abnormalities found within this area may reflect disorders of the structures involved or within other body systems.

Head

The skull provides protection and support for the underlying organs. The skull comprises the frontal, temporal, parietal, and occipital bones (see Figure 6-1). The area in which the individual bones meet is a called a fissure. The eyes are located within an opening in the anterior skull referred to as the orbit. The zygomatic arch is located below the eyes, between the temporal bone and the cheekbone. When discussing an anatomic area on the head, the underlying bony structures are utilized to name the area.

Hair is an extension of the epithelium on the head. The individual hair is a keratinized, stratified, multilayered squamous epithelium. Hair has a three-staged growth cycle—anagen, catagen, and telogen. The anagen phase is the active growth phase. The longer this stage lasts, the faster the hair will grow. At any given time, about 85% of the hair on the head is in this stage. The catagen

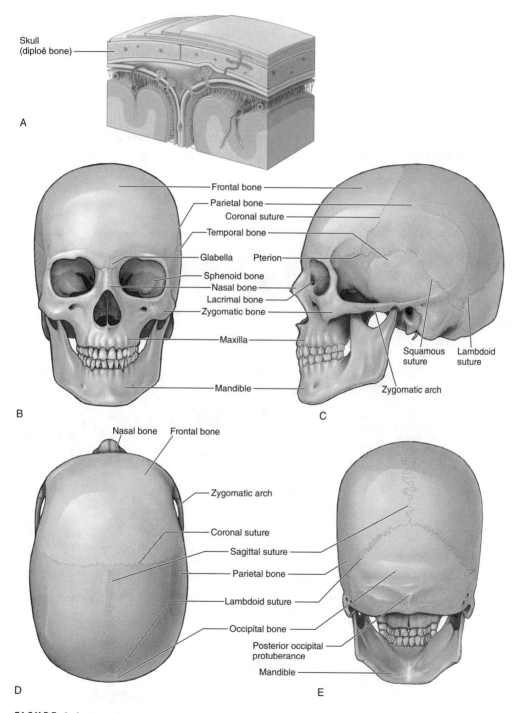

FIGURE 6-1 • Anatomy of the skull.
(Reproduced with permission from Morton DA, Foreman KB, Albertine KH: *The Big Picture: Gross Anatomy.* New York, NY: McGraw-Hill; 2011. Figure 15-2.)

phase is a transitional or resting phase. The telogen phase is a dormant phase. Hair is shed during this phase when a new hair strand pushes the older strand out of the follicle. All three stages occur simultaneously, with different hair in different stages. Hair grows at about 0.5 inch per month.

Eye

The anterior most structure of the eye is the cornea (see Figure 6-2). The pupil allows for light and visual images to travel toward the optic disc. Surrounding

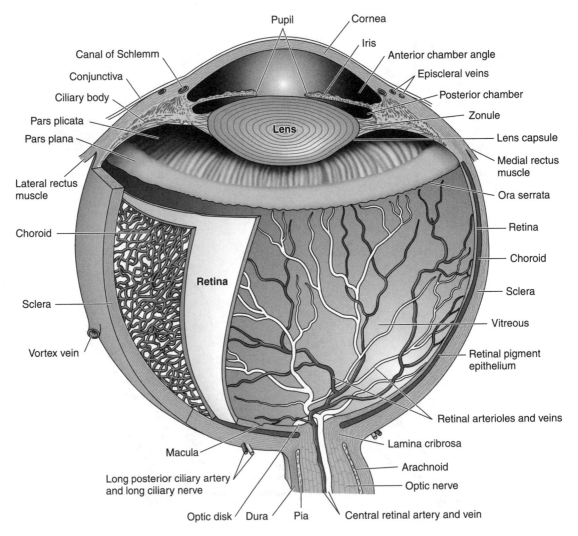

FIGURE 6-2 • Anatomy of the eye.
(Reproduced with permission from Riordan-Eva P, Cunningham E: *Vaughan & Asbury's General Ophthalmology*, 18th edition. New York, NY: McGraw-Hill; 2011. Figure 1-7.)

the pupil is the iris, or colored part of the eye. The white of the eye is the sclera. Behind the iris is the anterior chamber. This chamber is filled with aqueous humor (which has a watery consistency), which is constantly being produced, flushed through the anterior chamber, and drained through the canal of Schlemm. The eyeball is divided into anterior and posterior chambers by the crystalline lens. The posterior chamber is much larger than the anterior chamber and is filled with vitreous humor (which has a gelatinous consistency), and is not regenerated. The retina is found on the posterior surface of the eye and has a sensory layer and an underlying vascular layer. The optic disc is found on the retina. Arteries and veins originate at the optic disc and travel toward four quadrants of the retina. The fovea is the point of central vision and is surrounded by the macula.

Six muscles control the movement of the eyeball and are referred to as the extraocular muscles. There are four basic cardinal directions of eye movement—up, down, right, and left. Cranial nerves III, IV, and VI control the eye movements.

There are external structures present to provide protection to the eye. The upper and lower lids and eyelashes help keep foreign bodies out of the eye as well as keep the eye moist. The innermost area of the eye is the medial canthus. The outer portion of the eye is the lateral canthus. The upper lid normally covers the upper edge of the iris. The iris is the colored part of the eye. Centrally located within the iris is the pupil.

Ear

The ears are located on either sides of the head. The outer ear is positioned and shaped to help collect sound waves from the environment. The auricle or pinna is the external ear structure. It comprises cartilage and skin. The outer curvature of the ear is the helix; the smaller, inner curvature is the antihelix. The lower, soft part of the external ear is the lobe or lobule. The anterior most area of the external ear is the tragus. The ear canal begins at the external ear and ends at the tympanic membrane (see Figure 6-3). The canal is lined with skin, and has many nerve fibers and ceruminous glands. These glands produce cerumen, commonly referred to as earwax.

The middle ear begins at the tympanic membrane and ends at the oval window. A healthy ear drum should be pearly-gray color and reflect light. Three small ossicles, the malleus, incus, and stapes, are located internal to the tympanic membrane and vibrate in response to sound. The eustachian tube is a small canal that connects the middle ear and the pharynx, or throat. This canal

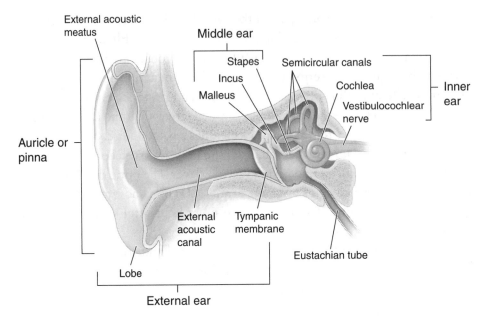

FIGURE 6-3 • Anatomy of the ear.
(Reproduced with permission from Longo DL, Fauci AS, Kasper DL, et al: *Harrison's Online*, 18th edition. New York, NY: McGraw-Hill; 2011. Figure 30-1A.)

allows for drainage from the middle ear and helps to equalize pressure within the middle ear.

The inner ear begins with the oval window and includes the cochlea and semicircular canals. Very small fibers (villa) are found within the inner ear and respond to subtle movements of the fluid contained here. The inner ear is integral to our senses of hearing and balance.

Sound waves are transmitted from the environment, collected by the auricle, travel through the ear canal, and cause vibration of the tympanic membrane. The vibration of the tympanic membrane causes vibration of the ossicles that will transmit the vibration to the fluid-filled cochlea. The villi within the cochlea will pick up the vibration of the fluid and transmit the signal to the acoustic (or auditory) nerve that transmits the signal to the brain.

Nose

The upper portion or bridge of the nose is supported by the nasal bones. The nasal bones support approximately the upper one-third of the nose. The lower portion of the nose is formed by cartilage. The overlying skin is thicker at the bridge and at the tip of the nose and is more delicate in the midsection of the nose.

The nasal mucosa is moist and pinkish-red in color, slightly darker than the oral mucosa. Ridges within the mucosa create turbinates that help to moisten and filter the air.

The sinuses are lined with mucous membranes and create air-filled spaces that serve to lighten the weight of the skull and give resonance to the voice. Consider the change in your own voice when you have sinus congestion due to a cold. Sinuses are located bilaterally in the frontal area (in the lower forehead, over the eyes), maxillary area (in the cheekbone area, under the eyes), ethmoid area (between the eyes, near the bridge of the nose), and the sphenoid area (between the eyes, behind the nasal cavity).

Mouth

The oral mucosa is pink and moist. The roof of the mouth comprises the hard palate (anteriorly) and soft palate (posteriorly).

The tongue comprises several muscles. The base of the tongue is attached to the floor of the mouth. The anterior most portion of the tongue is attached to the floor of the mouth by the frenulum. The underside of the tongue is smooth. The top surface of the tongue is covered with papillae, which contain the taste buds. The taste buds help us to identify sweet, salty, sour, and bitter taste. The anterior portion of the tongue senses sweet and salty taste. The lateral portions of the tongue sense sour taste. The posterior portion of the tongue senses bitter taste.

Primary teeth begin to break through the gums between 6 and 12 months of age. There are 20 primary teeth. Permanent teeth will force out the primary teeth starting at about the age of 5 or 6 years. This process is typically complete by the age of 12 or 13 years. There are 28 permanent teeth. During the late teenage years, four more teeth emerge at the back of the mouth, the wisdom teeth, bringing the total count to 32. The crown of the tooth is visible above the gum line. The shiny surface of the visible portion of the tooth is the enamel. The enamel protects the underlying tooth structures. Under the enamel the tooth is composed of dentin. The innermost structure is the pulp. Nerve fibers and blood supply are present within the pulp. The root of the tooth is made of cementum and anchors the tooth in place.

The front four teeth (top and bottom) are incisors. The next tooth on each side of the top and bottom are somewhat pointier and are the canine teeth. Next to the canine teeth are the bicuspids. There are eight bicuspid teeth, two on top and two on bottom on each side. Farther back in the mouth are the molars. The wisdom teeth are the most posterior teeth. Thirty-two teeth are seen, if all adult teeth are present.

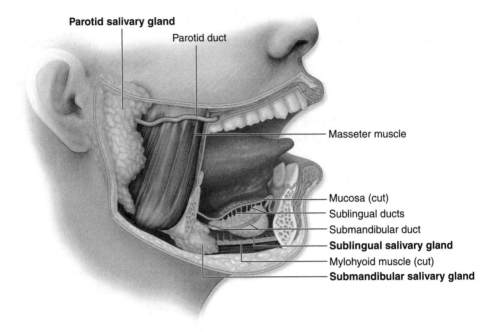

Parotid salivary gland
Parotid duct
Masseter muscle
Mucosa (cut)
Sublingual ducts
Submandibular duct
Sublingual salivary gland
Mylohyoid muscle (cut)
Submandibular salivary gland

FIGURE 6-4 ·
(Reproduced with permission from Mescher AL: *Junqueira's Basic Histology: Text & Atlas*, 12ᵗʰ edition. New York, NY: McGraw-Hill; 2010. Figure 16-1.)

The major salivary glands are the parotid, submandibular, and sublingual glands (see Figure 6-4). These glands are located bilaterally and secrete saliva into the mouth. The openings of the parotid salivary gland ducts can be found on the inner cheek, near the upper molars bilaterally. The openings of the sub-mandibular and sublingual gland ducts open to the floor of the mouth lateral to the frenulum bilaterally.

Throat

The mucosa of the oropharynx is a continuation of the oral mucosa and should be pink and moist. The uvula is found at the roof of the mouth and should be midline.

The palatine tonsils are found laterally in the pharynx, between the anterior and posterior pillars (see Figure 6-5). The tonsils may be fairly prominent in children and adolescents, and naturally get smaller as people age.

Neck

The sternocleidomastoid muscles are located bilaterally and attach to the manubrium of the sternum and the clavicles on the lower end, and the mastoid

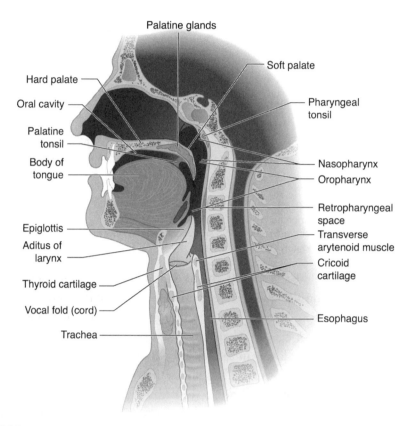

FIGURE 6-5 • Airway anatomy.
(Reproduced with permission from Tintinalli JE, Stapczynski JS, MA OJ et al: *Tintinalli's Emergency Medicine: A Comprehensive Study Guide*, 7th edition. New York, NY: McGraw-Hill; 2011. Figure 28-2.)

area and lower area of the occipital bones on the higher end. The trapezius muscle attaches to the scapula and thoracic vertebrae on the lower end and the occipital bone on the higher end. For landmarking purposes, the neck is divided into an anterior triangle and a posterior triangle. The anterior triangle is bordered by the mandible, the sternocleidomastoid muscle, and the midline of the anterior neck. The posterior triangle is bordered by the sternocleidomastoid muscle, the trapezius muscle, and the clavicle. Asking the patient to turn their head to one side makes the sternocleidomastoid muscle easier to locate.

There are several chains of cervical lymph nodes (see Figure 6-6). The preauricular node is located anterior to the tragus. The posterior auricular nodes are located behind the external ear, slightly above the mastoid process. The occipital nodes are found behind the sternocleidomastoid muscle and in front of the trapezius muscle, high in the posterior triangle of the neck. The tonsilar nodes are located behind the angle of the mandible. The anterior cervical chain

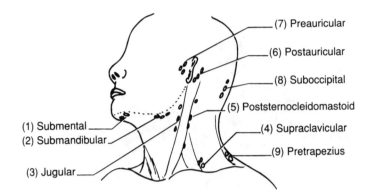

FIGURE 6-6 • Cervical lymph nodes.
(Reproduced with permission from LeBlond RF, DeGowin RL, Brown DD: *DeGowin's Diagnostic Examination*, 9th edition. New York, NY: McGraw-Hill; 2008. Figure 5-1.)

is located anterior to the sternocleidomastoid muscle, moving down and slightly anterior from the tonsilar node. The superficial cervical chain is located along the midposterior area of the sternocleidomastoid muscle, in the upper area of the neck. The posterior cervical chain is located posterior to the sternocleido-mastoid muscle, slightly lower in the neck. Following this line down, you will come to the supraclavicular or scalene nodes that are located posterior to the medial clavicles. The submandibular (or submaxillary) nodes are located beneath and medial to the lateral area of the mandible. The submental node is located behind the bony area of the chin.

The thyroid gland is an endocrine gland, which means the gland secretes hormones directly into the blood stream. The gland is butterfly shaped and located in the anterior neck and wraps around the front portion of the trachea (see Figure 6-7). The gland has a right and a left side (or "wings") that are connected by a central isthmus. The isthmus is located just below the Adam's apple (prominence made by the thyroid cartilage). Enlargement of the thyroid gland is called a goiter.

Subjective Information

Interview

During the interview process, focus should be on identifying any prior history or risk factors that would help in determining the cause of any symptoms that the patient may be experiencing.

Ask the patient about the history or injuries that would affect the head and neck area. For prior history, elicit the diagnosis (if known), the time frame, the

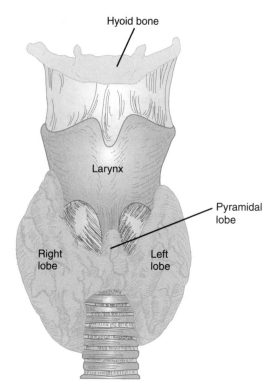

FIGURE 6-7 • Thyroid gland.
(Reproduced with permission from Barrett KE, Barman SM, Boltano S, et al: *Ganong's Review of Medical Physiology,* 24th edition. New York, NY: McGraw-Hill; 2012. Figure 19-1.)

treatment rendered, and its result. For injuries to the head, ask if there was any loss of consciousness, concussion, open wounds, or lingering symptoms.

Review of Systems (ROS)

Head

Ask the patient about chronic or current symptoms, such as headaches, or injuries to the head. If the patient experiences chronic headaches, it is important to determine the frequency, intensity, triggers, usual current treatments and their effectiveness, and any associated symptoms. Ask about any changes in headache with cough, Valsalva maneuver, or position changes. The headache pattern may be indicative of a tension headache, migraine, sinusitis, or space-occupying lesion within the skull. Nausea and/or vomiting may be associated with migraine headache, increased intracranial pressure (ICP), or infection. Concerning symptoms in need of rapid evaluation would include the onset of headaches after the age of 50 years; headache described as the "worst headache in my life";

significantly elevated blood pressure; signs of infection; or associated neurologic deficits.

Eye

Determine the patient's normal vision and any deviation from that. Blurring may be transient or constant. Loss of visual acuity may be a result of aging or from a systemic disease, such as diabetes mellitus. Double vision may be the result of a head injury, mass, or systemic disease, such as multiple sclerosis. Loss of all or part of the vision may be due to a stroke, migraine, or retinal detachment. Determine if the loss was sudden or gradual and if there is any associated pain. Ask about the presence of discharge or crusting. Discharge from the eye may be due to allergy, conjunctivitis, or other infectious causes. Crusting results from the drying of secretions along the lash line. Ask about any flecks in the visual field. Determine if they are stationary (scotomas), which may be reflect damage to the retina or optic nerve, or if they move (floaters), which likely represent vitreous changes. Ask about any pain in the eye or surrounding structures. Pain in the eye may be due to a minor irritation, trauma to the eye, or other pathology.

Ear

Determine the degree of the patient's normal hearing. Ask if the patient notes any difficulty understanding what is being said around them. If there is any difficulty, determine if it occurs when there is a lot of background noise, as in a crowded room, or if there are certain levels of sound that are more difficult, such as high-pitched versus low-pitched sounds. Ask about tinnitus. Tinnitus (ringing or buzzing) in the ears may be due to head trauma, damage to the acoustic nerve, or a result of exposure to loud noises. Ask about discharge from the ear. Discharge from the ear may be due to normal cerumen production, infection, trauma, or damage to the tympanic membrane. Ask about changes in or difficulty with balance. Loss of balance may be due to a problem within the inner ear or a neurologic disorder. Vertigo is the sensation of spinning. The patient may describe that the room is spinning or that they feel as if they are moving. This is typically due to an abnormality within the inner ear labyrinth, cranial nerve VIII, or lesions within the brain. Hearing loss, vertigo, and tinnitus are suggestive of Ménière's disease.

Nose

Ask about any congestion or nasal discharge. Congestion may be due to swelling of the nasal mucosa seen in colds, allergies, or due to tumor or a foreign body.

Nasal discharge is called rhinorrhea. Allergies and colds are common causes of nasal congestion and discharge. If the patient is experiencing any nasal discharge, ask about the amount and the color, the duration of the rhinorrhea, and any associated symptoms. Ask about the presence of nosebleeds or epistaxis. The most common reason for nosebleeds is self-injury (picking). Other considerations with nosebleeds would be chronic allergies, nasal exposure to drugs, trauma, a clotting disorder, or an excessive level of anticoagulation. Ask about any change in the patient's sense of smell.

Mouth

Ask about pain or any lesions in the mouth. Lesions may be from benign causes such as aphthous ulcers or a more serious condition such as cancer. Ask about color changes. A thick, white, adherent membrane may be indicative of candida infection. This may be an indicator of immune compromise in adults. Ask about bleeding gums. Bleeding may indicate dental problems or an underlying bleeding disorder.

Throat/Neck

Ask about throat irritation or sore throats. A sore throat may be due to a self-limited viral illness, bacterial infection, postnasal drip, allergies, environmental exposure, or gastric acid reflux. Ask about changes in the voice. Laryngitis may be a self-limited result of a cough or cold, or more chronic in nature due to smoking, allergies, voice overuse, or vocal cord polyps. Ask about swollen glands or lymph nodes. Swollen, tender lymph nodes may be associated with a local infection or systemic disease. Ask about any thyroid enlargement or goiter. Normal function of the thyroid regulates metabolism. Ask the patient about signs of overactive thyroid function: weight loss, heat intolerance, palpitations; and signs of hypoactive thyroid function: weight gain, cold intolerance, decreased sweating.

Risk Factors Related to the System

Certain diseases increase the risk for end-organ damage affecting the head, eyes, ears, nose, and throat (HEENT) areas. Diabetes or hypertension increases the risk of retinal pathology. Diabetes also increases the risks for oral problems, including dryness, cavity formation, and gum disease.

Some patients have significant occupational exposures that increase the risk for HEENT problems. Protective head gear is recommended when the chance of head injury is increased. Sports participation (football, lacrosse, etc) and certain professions require protection to the head. Protective eyewear is recommended if there is any potential for projectiles or chemical splashing. Long-term exposure to noise increases the chance of hearing loss. Repeated exposure to loud noise (power tools or equipment, weapons, loud music) will also accelerate the normal age-related hearing loss.

Risk Evaluation

Questioning the patient about occupation, lifestyle, recreational activities, exposures, systemic diseases, and medications helps in identifying those with increased risk for abnormalities or changes in the HEENT areas.

Visual changes are common as people age. Refractive errors, glaucoma, cataract formation, and macular degeneration are more common in older patients. Glaucoma is the leading cause of blindness in African Americans. Visual loss related to glaucoma typically begins with loss of peripheral vision. Many with glaucoma are unaware that they have the disorder. Risk factors for glaucoma include being African American, over the age of 65 years, having a family history of glaucoma, having diabetes, or having myopia (being near-sighted).

> **ALERT**
>
> Patients with either diabetes or hypertension have an increased risk of developing retinopathy. Vascular changes increase the risk for hemorrhage or leaking into the retinal tissue. The early stages of diabetic retinopathy are nonproliferative, the vessel walls leak, and there may be some visual distortion. Proliferative retinopathy occurs later as new vessels form. These vessels may not be structurally sound and may result in bleeding. Neovascularization is the formation of new microvascular networks. Angiogenesis is the growth of new shoots from existing blood vessels. Exudate formation is also increased in these patients.

Presbyopia is a normal physiologic change in the eye that typically occurs after the age of 40 years. A decrease in the elasticity of the lens results in decreased ability to focus on near objects. This is most notable when reading small print. Items with small print may need to be held at a farther distance in order to focus. Glasses that magnify help with the clarity of small print.

The leading cause of visual loss in older patients is macular degeneration. Since the macula is the area that allows clarity of central vision, damage to the macula results in problems with driving, reading, facial recognition, or small details such as those needed for crafts or minor home repairs. There is increased risk of developing macular degeneration when there is a family history, the patient is Caucasian, or there is a history of smoking.

Hearing loss is also more common as people age. Handheld audiometers can be effective for screening for hearing loss. There is an increased risk of hearing loss with a family history, infections (meningitis, rubella, syphilis), and noise exposure (loud music, machinery, gunfire). As people age, there is increased difficulty in perceiving certain tones. The greater the length of time (history) of exposure to loud noise, the more pronounced the hearing loss. The hearing loss associated with aging is called presbycusis.

Gingivitis and periodontal disease are commonly found in the adult population. Lack of access to dental care and exposure to acidic and sugary foods contribute to the prevalence. Oral cancer risk increases with the use of tobacco (both smoking and chewing) and excess alcohol intake. Assess for presence of ulcerations or leukoplakia. Proper fit of dentures is necessary to maintain adequate nutrition.

Exposure to tobacco increases the risk of developing laryngeal or pharyngeal (as well as other) cancers. Human papillomavirus is associated with an increased risk of oropharyngeal cancers. This is more common in men than women, and in non-Hispanic Caucasians or African Americans.

Objective Information

Equipment Needed

In addition to adequate light, you will need a penlight, ophthalmoscope, cotton, otoscope, tongue depressor, and gloves. A Snellen chart and a Jaeger chart are needed to assess visual acuity.

Assessment Techniques

In order to thoroughly examine the head and neck area, you need to utilize inspection, palpation, percussion, and auscultation.

Physical Examination

Inspect

Head: Examine the hair distribution on the scalp. Note the amount, distribution, and texture of hair, any areas of loss, presence of dandruff or nits (eggs of lice).

Note the skin color, changes in pigmentation, texture, or any lesions. Assess the underlying skin on the scalp for any abnormalities, such as lumps, redness, or lesions. Note the overall shape and size of the skull. Ask the patient to raise their eyebrows, puff out their cheeks, smile, and show their teeth. This will evaluate cranial nerve VII. Note the symmetry of facial features and expressions. Note any swelling, redness, or tics. Check for the presence of any infestation, such as lice. Make sure to move some of the hair to look underneath.

Eye: Note the eye structures—the lids, sclera, iris, pupils, palpebral fissures, and conjunctiva. Note any discharge, lesions, or color alterations. Check for pupillary reaction to light with a penlight. The pupil that has the light shining toward it should constrict. This is a direct response. The other pupil should also constrict. This is a consensual response. Pupillary reactions evaluate cranial nerve II. Evaluate extraocular movements by asking the patient to follow your finger as you go through the six cardinal positions of gaze. Test convergence by asking the patient to follow your finger as you move it toward their face in a midline position. Alignment of the eyes can be tested by shining a light directed between the eyes and noting the location of the light reflex (seen as a small white spot) on each eye (see Figure 6-8). The light reflex should be located in the same place on both eyes. Visual acuity is measured with a Snellen chart

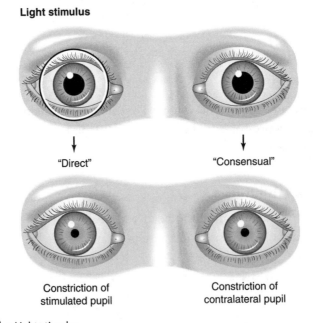

Light stimulus

"Direct"   "Consensual"

Constriction of
stimulated pupil

Constriction of
contralateral pupil

FIGURE 6-8 • Light stimulus.
(Reproduced with permission from Riordan-Eva P, Cunningham E: *Vaughan & Asbury's General Ophthalmology*, 18th edition. New York, NY: McGraw-Hill; 2011. Figure 14-31.)

(from 20 feet) or a Jaeger chart (from 14 inches). This assesses cranial nerve II. The ability to differentiate colors (color vision) can be tested with an Ishihara color test.

Ophthalmoscope: An ophthalmoscope allows visualization of the inner structures of the eye. It can be focused to adjust for refractive errors of the patient or the healthcare provider. You will also have the option of several different types of light for examination. There will be a large circular white light, a small circular white light, a skinny rectangular-shaped light (for slit lamp examination), a circular white light with a superimposed grid (to aid in describing location of abnormalities), and in many cases a green or blue light. When you are examining the patient's right eye, you will use your right eye. You will use your left eye when examining the patient's left eye. Changing your viewpoint in this way prevents you from coming nose to nose with the patient as you get closer for a better view. The patient should be comfortably seated for the examination. You will position yourself to the side of the patient. Look through the ophthalmoscope while holding it in front of your examining eye. Make sure the light is directed toward the patient and not toward you. Line up the light from the ophthalmoscope with the patient's pupil. You should see the reflection of the retina, which makes the pupil appear bright and it should appear as a pinkish-red color. This is called a red reflex. Patients who have different eye colors (blue vs. brown, etc) will have red reflexes that are slightly different in color. Once you have located the red reflex, you will follow it inward toward the patient. Think of the pupil as a keyhole that you are looking through. It is a small opening and you will need to move to allow visualization of different areas within the eye while maintaining visual alignment with the pupil. As you are moving in toward the patient, it is helpful to place your hand on their shoulder or forehead to help you judge distance. This should prevent you from bumping into the patient during the examination when you are focused on what you are seeing through the ophthalmoscope. Once you have moved in toward the patient, you should locate the optic disc. This is a creamy white circular area found toward the nasal side of the retina. You should see vessels coming from that area. The vessels are paired (artery and vein) and travel in four different directions: upward toward the nasal side, upward toward the temporal side, downward toward the nasal side, and downward toward the temporal side. The vessels become narrower as they travel away from the optic disc. The arteries are brighter in color and have a light reflex. You should also examine the fovea (the area of the retina responsible for central vision). You will need to move to the other side to examine the other eye and repeat the process. This examination takes practice for comfort and proficiency.

Ear: Begin by visually examining the external ear structures. Check for placement of pinna, presence of any lesions, or deformities. Place a protective cover on the tip of the otoscope. Use the otoscope to provide light and magnification of the visible structures within the ear canal. The ear canal needs to be straightened out to allow for better visualization. In a child, the pinna should be gently pulled down and back. In an adult, the pinna should be gently pulled up and back. Be careful while inserting the tip of the otoscope into the ear, as there are many nerve fibers within the ear canal. You do not want to hurt the patient during the examination. Some patients may not mention if your examination is causing pain, so be aware of the patient's body language. When examining children or those with altered cognitive status, it is helpful to brace the side of your hand against their head to prevent injury if the patient moves unexpectedly. Examine the ear canal. You may see cerumen (wax) within the ear canal. You should be able to see the tympanic membrane (or eardrum) which has a pearly-gray color. There will be a reflection of the light (called a cone of light) shining on the tympanic membrane (see Figure 6-9). This cone of light begins at the center of the tympanic membrane (near the umbo) and shines downward and forward. The right tympanic membrane will have a cone of light shining toward 5 O'clock, and the left ear will have the cone of light shining toward 7 O'clock.

Assess hearing with a whisper test. Stand behind and to the side of the patient and whisper a two- or three-syllable word. A ticking watch can also be used to evaluate hearing. Tuning fork tests may be used to differentiate a conductive hearing loss from a sensory hearing loss. A Weber test uses a vibrating tuning fork with the handle placed against the bone in the middle of the head.

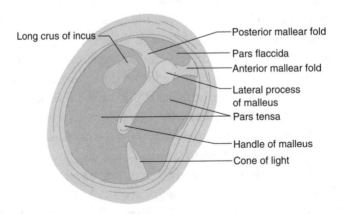

FIGURE 6-9 • Right tympanic membrane, as seen through an otoscope.
(Reproduced with permission from Tintinalli JE, Stapczynski JS, MA OJ et al: *Tintinalli's Emergency Medicine: A Comprehensive Study Guide*, 7th edition. New York, NY: McGraw-Hill; 2011. Figure 237-2.)

Ask the patient which ear hears a louder sound. In a conductive hearing loss, the sound that is transmitted through the bone will be perceived as louder in the affected ear, whereas a sensorineural hearing loss will cause the sound to be perceived as louder in the nonaffected ear. A Rinne test determines whether air conduction is longer than bone conduction of sound. Place the handle of a vibrating tuning fork on the mastoid process behind the ear and ask the patient to tell you when they no longer hear the sound. Move the tuning fork so that the tines are next to the patient's ear and ask the patient to let you know when the sound stops. Some patients are more sensitive to the sound made by the tuning fork—in this case, move the tuning fork further away from the ear. Normally, air conduction is longer than bone conduction and is documented as AC>BC. Assessment of hearing evaluates cranial nerve VIII.

Nose: Look at the outer structures of the nose, the alignment, and the condition of the skin. Using a light source, inspect the nasal mucosa and the nasal septum for color, moisture, discharge, and lesions or perforations.

Mouth: Look at the lips. Look for cracking or fissures at the corners of the mouth. Inspect the mucosa for color and moisture. Note any lesions or areas of irritation. Aphthous ulcers (canker sores) have a well-demarcated edge and a white or yellow surface surrounded by an erythematous (reddened) base, and may be painful to touch. Note the number and condition of the teeth. An adult should have 32 teeth, including the wisdom teeth. The enamel of the teeth should be white, intact, and without decay. Ask the patient to stick out their tongue. This assesses cranial nerve XII.

Throat: By using an external light source (like a penlight), inspect the pharynx. The mucosa should appear pink and moist. Ask the patient to say "aahhhh." This will raise the soft palate, allowing better visualization of the posterior oropharynx (back of the throat). Rising of the soft palate evaluates cranial nerves IX and X. The uvula should remain in midline as the soft palate rises. Deviation of the uvula from midline may indicate a problem affecting cranial nerve X.

Neck: Inspect the neck for any asymmetry. The trachea should be midline. There should not be any visible masses. There should be smooth, unlimited range of motion. The Adam's apple rises when the patient swallows.

Palpate

Head: Feel for normal skull structures. Check for any areas of depression or presence of irregular bone structure. Note any areas of tenderness on palpation. Press over the sinus areas (frontal and maxillary) bilaterally to determine if there is any tenderness on palpation.

Eye: The closed lid of the eye may be gently palpated to check for tenderness. The lid margins may be palpated to assess any abnormalities (such as a stye). The bony orbits can be palpated for tenderness. A corneal reflex can be assessed by gently touching a wisp of cotton to the cornea. This assesses cranial nerves V and VII. Make sure the patient is not wearing contact lenses when testing. The normal response is blinking. People who normally wear contact lenses will have less of a response.

Ear: Palpate the external ear structures, the pinna, the lobe, and the tragus for abnormalities or tenderness. Gently tug on the pinna to determine if there is any discomfort on movement.

Nose: You can palpate the nose to determine if there is any tenderness. Be aware of the underlying anatomy—whether you are palpating over bone, cartilage, or soft tissue.

Mouth: Wear gloves for palpation of oral structures. Feel for any areas of induration or masses. Palpate the gums, tongue, and floor of the mouth. You can assess perception of taste in the different areas of the tongue. This will evaluate cranial nerve IX.

Throat: The throat is generally not palpated. You may need to check a gag reflex by gently touching a tongue depressor against the posterior pharynx. Assessment of a gag reflex evaluates cranial nerve IX.

Neck: Locate the appropriate anatomic landmarks of the neck. The trachea should be midline. You will find the thyroid and hyoid cartilage encircling the trachea. The thyroid gland wraps around the anterior aspect of the trachea. It is narrow over the anterior most portion and widens out (like wings) on either side. Asking the patient to swallow helps to locate the proper area to examine. Gentle palpation of the thyroid can isolate nodules or determine if there is a disparity in the sizes of each lobe. You can gently push the thyroid toward one side (mildly displacing the trachea) to allow for better palpation.

Gentle palpation over the cervical node chains can detect enlargement, change in texture, or tenderness. Systematically approach the chains of the lymph nodes, so that all chains are assessed.

Percuss

Head: Gently tap the skin over the frontal and maxillary sinus areas to assess for tenderness.

Auscultate

Head: Use the stethoscope to listen over the temporal artery. Note any bruit.

Neck: Use both the bell and diaphragm of the stethoscope to listen over the carotid arteries. Note the presence of any bruits. Different sources recommend use of the bell or use of the diaphragm for carotid bruit assessment. The bell will transmit low-frequency sounds better, whereas the diaphragm will transmit higher frequency sounds better. A bruit typically has a higher frequency sound (diaphragm), since the blood flow tends to be fast and turbulent. However, if there is sufficient narrowing of the vessel, the blood flow may be diminished which could result in a lower frequency sound (bell).

Expected Findings

Head

The head should be symmetrical without any signs of injury or malformation. Both inspection and palpation of the skull should demonstrate a solid structure without areas of depression or unnatural movement. Hair distribution should be symmetric without areas of alopecia (loss). There should not be any nits or lice noted.

Eye/Vision

You should see symmetry of structures. Conjunctiva should be clear, moist, and without discharge. Pupils should constrict in response to light. A light reflected off the cornea (light reflex) should have the reflection located at the same point on both eyes. The patient should be able to follow the object when testing extraocular movements. Testing for convergence should reveal that the eyes follow the object as it moves closer, turning inward. The vision should be 20/20, which means that the patient can read at a distance of 20 feet what the average person can read at a distance of 20 feet. This is commonly checked with a Snellen chart, from a distance of 20 feet.

Ear/Hearing

The outer ear should have intact skin and be symmetrically equal. There should be no tenderness on palpation. You should be able to move the patient's outer ear without pain. The auditory canal should be clear. A scant amount of cerumen may be present and is considered normal. The tympanic membrane should be intact, have a pearly-gray color and have a bright light reflex (in a downward, anterior direction from the center). You should be able to visualize the umbo of the malleolus behind the tympanic membrane. The patient should be able to hear and understand the spoken word.

Throat/Speech

The mucous membranes should be pink and moist, without exudate. The tonsils (if present) should be between the anterior and posterior pillars.

Mouth/Taste

The mucous membranes should be pink and moist. The teeth should be intact without signs of cavity or decay. There should be no lesions or erosions. The salivary duct openings should be without inflammation.

Neck

The neck should appear symmetrical, with a midline trachea. Palpation should not produce pain. The cervical lymph nodes should be smooth, mobile, non-tender, and not enlarged. The thyroid should have a smooth, rubbery consistency. The carotid pulses should be strong and equal bilaterally. There should not be any bruit detected.

Abnormal Findings

Head

Asymmetry or obvious signs of trauma or recent injury.

Eye/Vision

The structures of the eye should be without signs of irritation, infection, or injury. Redness or drainage would be abnormal findings. A light source that reflects off the cornea in different locations (for example: midpupil on right and at the edge of the pupil on the left) indicates asymmetry of the eyes.

Ear/Hearing

Asymmetry of the outer ears may indicate a congenital defect or injury to one or both ears. Pain on movement or palpation of the outer ear may indicate infection or inflammation. Redness or swelling within the ear canal are abnormal findings. Drainage within the ear canal is abnormal and may indicate infection or perforation of the tympanic membrane. Cerumen that occludes the ear canal is excessive and should be removed. Absence of the light reflex on the tympanic membrane is abnormal. Scarring or a hole within the tympanic membrane is abnormal. Redness of the tympanic membrane with an intact light reflex may be a transient finding. If the light reflex is absent with a reddened tympanic membrane, fluid may be trapped within the middle ear, or an infection may be present. A patient that needs to have repetition of questions may have diminished hearing.

Throat/Speech

Reddened mucous membranes indicate irritation. Exudate may be present on the posterior pharynx or the tonsils. Enlarged tonsils indicate inflammation. Hoarseness or laryngitis may be indicative of a self-limited condition, such as a viral infection. Persistent laryngitis, lasting more than 3 weeks, may be indicative of gastroesophageal reflux, nerve damage, vocal cord polyps, exposure to inhaled irritants, overuse of the voice, smoking, or cancer.

Mouth/Taste

Redness indicates irritation. Missing, eroded, or poorly maintained teeth may indicate dental problems or systemic disorders. Lesions may indicate local or systemic disease.

Neck

Firm, tender, enlarged lymph nodes are abnormal. Tenderness may indicate inflammation. Enlarged, hard, nontender nodes may be indicative of cancer or other pathology. An uneven, asymmetrical thyroid, or presence of nodules are abnormal findings. A bruit indicates increased turbulence of blood flow, which may be due to plaque buildup within the artery.

Age-Related Changes

Pediatric

Children are not just small adults. It is important to be familiar with age-appropriate normal findings. The sense of touch is well developed in infants. Infants who are stimulated through touch (tactile) may not respond as expected to stimulation of the other senses.

Look at the general appearance of the head. Newborns may have an unusually shaped head for the first day or two of life due to molding of the head during vaginal birth. The bones of the skull are not fused in a neonate to allow for remodeling necessary for birth. The spaces between the bones will close to create a hard skull that will protect the brain. The posterior fontanel closes by about 2 months of age and the anterior fontanel closes between 10 and 18 months. Prior to closing, fontanels may bulge with increased intracranial pressure(ICP) or may be depressed or sunken with dehydration. The head should be symmetrically shaped. Asymmetry may be indicative of sutures that have closed too quickly. Surgery may be needed to correct this abnormality.

Head circumference is measured using a flexible measuring tape in infants as part of a routine examination up until about 2 years of age. The circumference is checked at the largest part of the head, above the eyebrows and ears. Measurement is checked against age- and gender-specific ranges, and also compared with results from prior examinations. A larger than expected measurement may signal that there is excess growth, or the development of hydrocephalus (cerebrospinal fluid collecting within the skull). A measurement that is smaller than expected may indicate that the brain is not developing normally.

Look at the hair distribution on the scalp. Areas of hair loss (alopecia) may be indicative of local infection, hair pulling, or repeated (or prolonged) positioning of an infant in the same position. Check for lice or nits attached to the hair. Infestation is most common in school-aged children.

There should be a normal red reflex and blink reflex noted at the beginning of the neonatal period. A fundoscopic examination is performed as in an adult. Between 1 and 2 months of age, the infant should be able to follow a visual stimulus. As children become older, visual screening is performed. A chart with a capital letter E in varied sizes, with the opening facing in different directions or a chart with familiar pictures (house, star, tree, etc) is used to check visual acuity in preschool-aged children. A Snellen chart (varied letters in progressively smaller sizes) is used for school-aged children and older.

The eyes should be symmetrically located. Eyes that are set more narrowly or wider than expected may indicate a systemic disorder. A corneal light reflex should reflect light at the same point on both eyes. Ambylopia, or a "lazy eye," may signify that one of the muscles that control the eye is not having the same strength as the other muscles, causing the eye to be pulled toward (stronger) or away from (weaker) the affected muscle. Children with chronic allergies may develop "allergic shiners" or dark circles under the eyes.

Screening for hearing is performed periodically in children. Additional screening may be indicated if there are language delays or frequent ear infections.

Check for symmetry and the position of the ears, relative to the location of the eyes. Congenital anomalies may result in abnormal positioning of the ears.

Ear examinations (and other invasive procedures) should be performed toward the end of the encounter. In infants and young children, pull the auricle down and back to straighten the ear canal for otoscopic examination. In older children and adolescents, pull the ear up and back, as in adults.

Infants need to breathe through their noses. Check for patency of the nostrils, presence of discharge, swelling, or deviation of the septum. Nasal flaring may be noted in infants or children with respiratory difficulty. Children with chronic allergies may develop an "allergic salute," a line across the anterior nose that develops after repeatedly rubbing upward against the tip of the nose. Congenital anomalies may result in flattening of the nose or nasolabial folds.

Inspect the palate of a newborn for abnormalities, such as cleft palate. Check the tongue for appropriate movement. The frenulum that attaches the tongue to the floor of the mouth should allow for adequate movement of the tongue. Teeth begin to erupt at about 6 months of age. Primary teeth continue to erupt about once a month until there are 20 teeth. Check the teeth of adolescents for erosion of the enamel, which may indicate an eating disorder (from vomiting).

Hypertrophy of the tonsils is common in school-aged children and adolescents. Tonsils get smaller as people get older. The thyroid gland is not normally palpated in young children.

Geriatric

Loss of some subcutaneous fat in the temporal area is normal with aging.

Exposed skin areas, such as the head and neck, are common areas for skin changes, such as actinic keratosis and skin cancer.

Atrophy of the periorbital fat makes the eyes seem to have a sunken appearance. The pupils are typically smaller in older adults. Development of cataracts (opacity of the lens) is more common as people age. Relaxation of the tissues around the eyes may lead to entropion (the eyelid and lashes turn inward, or toward the cornea) or ectropion (the eyelid and lashes turn outward, away from the cornea). Tear production decreases with aging. Some patients will note that their eyes "water" due to atrophy of the tissues around the eye, which interferes with the normal flow of tears to the lacrimal duct. Arcus senilis is a gray-white line that develops at the edge of the iris in older patients and is not clinically significant. Drooping of the upper eyelid (ptosis) may result in visual impairment. Glaucoma is more common with aging.

Vision changes are typically noticed in people after 40 years of age. Difficulty with accommodation develops as the lens becomes less pliable and less able to focus at varied distances. This lack of accommodation is called presbyopia.

Difficulty with small print is often one of the first signs of presbyopia. Patients may note an increased sensitivity to glare. The ability to discriminate colors decreases with aging.

An increase in the amount and coarseness of hair within the ear canal may result in mild hearing loss or accumulation of cerumen within the ear canal. Hearing loss is more common as people age. Loss of higher tones usually occurs first. Patients with prolonged exposure to loud noise are more likely to have more pronounced hearing loss. The hearing loss that occurs as a normal part of aging is called presbycusis.

The interior of the mouth may be drier due to decreased salivation or side effects of medications. Dentures may become ill-fitting due to weight changes. Poorly fitting dentures may contribute to altered nutritional intake. The sensation of taste alters with aging. Loss of taste sensation can also contribute to altered nutritional intake. The ability to detect sweet taste is preserved the longest.

Cultural Considerations

You will notice some differences in facial structure and eye shape based on ethnicity.

There are no major cultural differences in risk, response to disease, or physical examination findings based on cultural differences.

CASE STUDY

Andy is a 76-year-old male who complains of dryness and irritation in his left eye. He notes that it constantly feels as if there is something in the eye and has also noted an increase in tearing in that eye. On examination you note that the lower lid of Andy's left eye appears to have turned inward with the lashes on, or very near to, the cornea.

REVIEW QUESTIONS

1. Taste buds are located on the tongue. You know that sweet taste is perceived on:
   A. the anterior portion of the tongue.
   B. the lateral portion of the tongue.
   C. the middle portion of the tongue.
   D. the posterior portion of the tongue.

2. **Aqueous humor has a watery consistency and fills the anterior chamber of the eye. This fluid is drained from the anterior chamber through the:**
   A. iris.
   B. canal of Schlemm.
   C. conjunctiva.
   D. cornea.

3. **The healthcare provider is using an otoscope to evaluate the tympanic membrane. Which of the following describes a normal finding?**
   A. A pearly-gray surface with a light reflex and a visible umbo.
   B. A pink surface with a small opening in the anterior lower quadrant and small air bubbles.
   C. A reddened bulging surface with visible vesicles.
   D. A dull gray surface with no light reflex.

4. **The preauricular cervical node is correctly palpated:**
   A. in the midline, just below the bony area of the chin.
   B. behind the external ear, slightly above the mastoid process.
   C. behind the sternocleidomastoid muscle.
   D. anterior to the tragus.

5. **The patient has a headache. Concerning symptoms in need of rapid evaluation would include:**
   A. multidecade history of migraine headaches.
   B. onset of headaches after the age of 20 years.
   C. associated systemic symptoms such as marked hypertension, fever, and malaise, or neurologic signs.
   D. headache onset and symptoms typical of other headache the patient has experienced for many years.

6. **Persistent laryngitis is defined as laryngitis that lasts for over:**
   A. 48 hours.
   B. 2 weeks.
   C. 3 weeks.
   D. 3 months.

7. **The leading cause of blindness in African Americans is:**
   A. cataracts.
   B. trauma.
   C. glaucoma.
   D. retinopathy.

8. **The healthcare provider is checking for pupillary reaction by shining a light into the patient's right eye. The left pupil constricts. This is known as:**

   A. direct response.

   B. consensual response.

   C. convergence.

   D. alignment.

9. **When performing an ophthalmoscopic examination of the patient's right eye, you position yourself on the right side of the patient and look through the ophthalmoscope and then:**

   A. see the optic disc.

   B. locate the lacrimal duct opening.

   C. locate the red reflex.

   D. compare the veins and arteries on the retina.

10. **When checking for a carotid bruit, you should use:**

    A. the bell of the stethoscope.

    B. the diaphragm of the stethoscope.

    C. a Doppler.

    D. both the bell and diaphragm of the stethoscope.

ANSWERS

1. A. The anterior portion of the tongue senses both sweet and salty taste; the lateral portions of the tongue sense sour and the posterior portion of the tongue senses bitter taste.

2. B. An aqueous humor fills the anterior chamber and is drained through the canal of Schlemm.

3. A. A normal tympanic membrane has a pearly-gray surface with a light reflex and a visible umbo.

4. D. The preauricular node is correctly palpated in front of the tragus.

5. C. Concerning symptoms in need of rapid evaluation would include the onset of symptoms after the age of 50 years; headaches described as the "worst headache of my life"; significantly elevated blood pressure; signs of infection; or associated neurologic deficits.

6. C. Persistent laryngitis lasts for more than 3 weeks.

7. C. The leading cause of blindness in African Americans is glaucoma.

8. B. A consensual pupillary response is seen when the contralateral pupil constricts when a light is shone on the pupil.

9. C. When performing an ophthalmoscopic examination, you position yourself to the side of the patient, look through the ophthalmoscope, and locate the red reflex.

10. D. When checking for a carotid bruit, you should use both the bell and the diaphragm of the stethoscope.

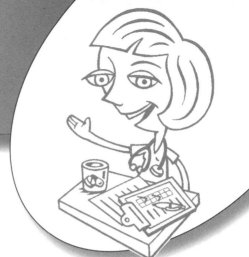

chapter 7

Assessment of the Respiratory System

LEARNING OBJECTIVES

After reviewing this chapter, the learner will be able to:

1. Identify important anatomic landmarks of the respiratory system.
2. Discuss the appropriate information to gather during an interview.
3. Demonstrate a physical assessment of the respiratory system.
4. List normal physical assessment findings.
5. Describe abnormal physical assessment findings.
6. Discuss the age-related differences related to the respiratory system.

KEYWORDS

Angle of Louis	Inspiration
Crackles	Intercostal spaces
Cricoid cartilage	Oblique fissure
Cyanosis	Sternum
Egophony	Trachea

Introduction

Normal function of the respiratory system provides oxygen for the entire body. Carbon dioxide is the end product of cellular metabolism within the body and is exhaled from the respiratory system. Changes in respiration may occur as part of a disease process or in response to alterations in other body systems, such as metabolic alkalosis.

Review of Anatomy and Physiology

The majority of the respiratory system is protected from damage or trauma by the bony structures, including the sternum (anteriorly), the vertebral column (posteriorly), and the ribcage. The sternum is divided into three sections: the manubrium (upper), the body (middle), and the xyphoid process (lower). A midline curve along the superior edge of the manubrium (the suprasternal notch) can be easily located by palpation. The sternal angle (or Angle of Louis) is the point where the manubrium and body of the sternum meet, and is located a couple of centimeters below the sternal notch (see Figure 7-1). This corresponds to the level of the second rib or intercostal space. There are 12 pairs of ribs that protect the lungs. Cartilage attaches the anterior ribs either directly to the sternum (ribs 1-7) or to the cartilage above (ribs 8 -10). The 11th and 12th ribs are free floating. The end of the 11th rib can be palpated laterally, whereas the 12th rib may be palpated along the back. Cartilage that is attached to the ribs is called costal cartilage. The spaces between the ribs are called intercostal spaces. You can locate things anatomically on the chest by counting the ribs and intercostal spaces either by working down after identification of the sternal angle or counting up from the 10th rib. Posteriorly, you can also use the vertebral bodies to landmark. Each rib is attached to a corresponding thoracic vertebra (the first rib attaches to the first thoracic vertebra or T1). The most

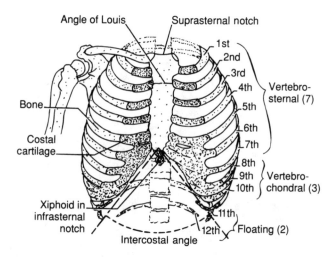

FIGURE 7-1 • Thoracic anatomy.
(Reproduced with permission from LeBlond RF, DeGowin RL, Brown DD: *DeGowin's Diagnostic Examination*, 9th edition. New York, NY: McGraw-Hill; 2008. Figure 8-1.)

prominent vertebral process is the seventh cervical vertebra or C7. This is easily located as it is the most prominent vertebral process noted when the patient flexes the neck (chin towards chest). Some individuals have two prominent vertebrae; in this case, the superior (upper) one is C7 and the inferior (lower) one is T1. You can also work up from the 12th rib. When the patient is sitting with their arms relaxed at their sides, the lower edge of the scapula is at the level of the seventh rib or intercostal space.

The respiratory system can be divided into the upper and lower airways. The upper airway includes the nasal passages, sinuses, pharynx, and larynx. The lower airway includes the trachea, bronchi, lungs, bronchioles, and alveoli (see Figure 7-2). Air is inhaled through the nasal passages and passes over the mucous membranes that line the nose and sinuses. The mucous membranes lining the nose, turbinates, and the sinuses help to humidify and adjust the temperature of the inspired air. Filtration of the air also occurs in the upper airways. Particulates (pollen, dust, etc) are removed from the air before it enters the lower airways.

The inhaled air passes through the pharynx, larynx, and trachea, and then bifurcates (or divides) into the right and left main stem bronchi. The right bronchus is straighter than the left. Due to the angle of the right main stem bronchus, it is more likely that patients who aspirate will have particles of aspiration (food, liquid, vomitus, etc) within the right lung. The level of bifurcation is approximately at the level of the Angle of Louis (or sternal angle). Posteriorly, this is approximately the level of the fourth thoracic vertebrae or T4.

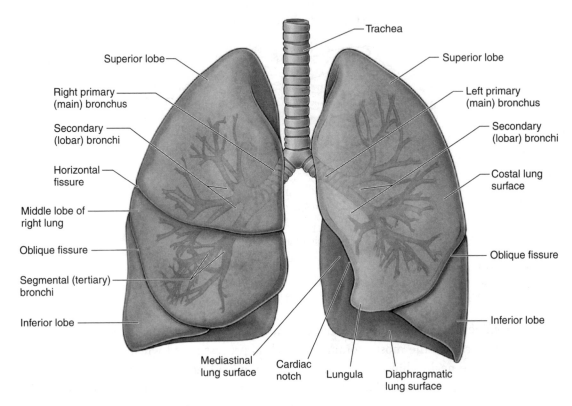

FIGURE 7-2 • Bronchial tree and lungs.
(Reproduced with permission from Morton DA, Foreman KB, Albertine KH: *The Big Picture: Gross Anatomy.* New York, NY: McGraw-Hill; 2011. Figure 3-2B.)

The lungs extend from above the clavicle to about the sixth rib anteriorly and the eighth rib in the midaxillary line. The lungs are divided into lobes, two on the left and three on the right. The upper lobe has greater presence along the anterior chest, whereas the lower lobe is better assessed along the posterior surface of the chest. The division between the upper and lower lobes is marked by an oblique fissure. This fissure extends from the level of the second thoracic vertebra (T2) to the level where the cartilage of the sixth rib attaches anteriorly. The horizontal fissure separates the right middle lobe from the upper lobe. This fissure is located from the fourth rib medially to the fifth rib laterally. When assessing the lungs, picture the underlying lobes. The right middle lobe can only be assessed from the anterior or lateral areas of the chest.

Gas exchange occurs within the alveoli. There is a large network of capillaries within the alveoli of the lungs (see Figure 7-3). The walls of the alveoli and pulmonary capillaries have semi-permeable membranes that allow for the diffusion of oxygen (O_2) and carbon dioxide (CO_2). There is a higher

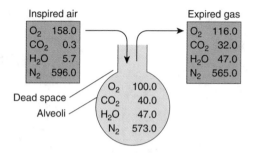

Inspired air

O_2	158.0
CO_2	0.3
H_2O	5.7
N_2	596.0

Expired gas

O_2	116.0
CO_2	32.0
H_2O	47.0
N_2	565.0

Dead space

Alveoli

O_2	100.0
CO_2	40.0
H_2O	47.0
N_2	573.0

FIGURE 7-3 • Representation of gas exchange in the lungs.
(Reproduced with permission from Barrett KE, Barman SM, Boltano S, et al: *Ganong's Review of Medical Physiology*, 24th edition. New York, NY: McGraw-Hill; 2012. Figure 34-15.)

concentration of oxygen within the inhaled air and a higher concentration of carbon dioxide in the blood flow that reaches the alveoli. These gases move from an area of higher concentration to an area of lower concentration. The oxygen-rich blood leaves the lungs and supplies the tissues of the body, where diffusion allows for the movement of oxygen from the high concentration within the circulation to the lower concentration of the body tissues. Carbon dioxide is released from the cells into the capillary circulation. It is transported to the lungs where the carbon dioxide crosses the alveolar membrane and will be exhaled.

Inspiration is an active process that involves the inspiratory muscles. The inspiratory muscles include the diaphragm and external intercostal muscles. During inspiration negative pressure is generated within the chest, which allows atmospheric air to enter the lungs. The nerves that supply the diaphragm originate in the cervical spinal column and the nerves in the thoracic spinal column supply the intercostal muscles. Expiration is the result of passive recoil of the lungs and the action of the rectus abdominus and internal intercostal muscles (see Figure 7-4).

Chemoreceptors are located centrally and peripherally and monitor the levels of oxygen, carbon dioxide, and hydrogen ions within the arterial circulation. The respiratory drive in healthy individuals is triggered when the carbon dioxide level ($PaCO_2$) within the arteries rises. The increased level will stimulate the respiratory center within the medulla oblongata and the pons, and will result in an increase in the respiratory rate and the depth of the respirations. A small percentage (up to 10%) of breathing control is thought to be controlled by the hypoxic respiratory drive. In this case, breathing is triggered by peripheral sensation of low oxygen levels. Patients with chronic respiratory disease, such as emphysema, will retain carbon dioxide. Over time their normal resting CO_2 levels will gradually increase, which can have an effect on their respiratory drive.

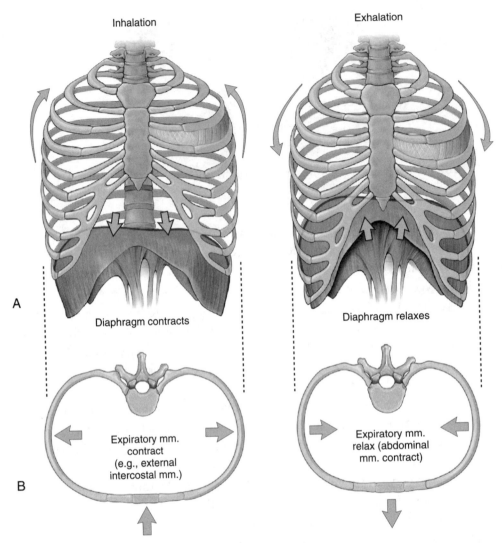

Inhalation

Exhalation

A

Diaphragm contracts

Diaphragm relaxes

B

Expiratory mm. contract (e.g., external intercostal mm.)

Expiratory mm. relax (abdominal mm. contract)

FIGURE 7-4 • Movements of the thoracic wall during inspiration and expiration in the anterior (A) and axial superior (B) views.
(Reproduced with permission from Morton DA, Foreman KB, Albertine KH: *The Big Picture: Gross Anatomy*. New York, NY: McGraw-Hill; 2011. Figure 3-4 A&B.)

Lower levels of oxygen are also detected by the peripheral chemoreceptors in these patients. There is some debate over how much impact the hypoxic respiratory drive actually has on an individual's respiratory status.

Breathing is normally an unconscious action. The presence of pain or alterations in body temperature can cause changes in respiration. Level of consciousness also impacts the depth and rate of breathing. Breathing can also be under voluntary control.

Airway resistance causes obstructive respiratory disease (emphysema) and loss of compliance is seen in restrictive disease (respiratory distress syndrome).

Subjective Information

Interview

Consider the patient's current condition when interviewing. Patients that are experiencing difficulty breathing will not be comfortable (or able) to answer a lot of questions. Asking questions that require 'need to know' and short answers may be necessary before the patient is stabilized. Other questions are best left until the patient is breathing more comfortably.

Review of Systems (ROS)

Shortness of breath is a subjective symptom. Any patient that experiences the sensation that they are having difficulty breathing or not getting enough air will likely have associated fear and anxiety. Ask the patient if they are experiencing shortness of breath. Also ask when the shortness of breath occurs. Is it present all the time, at a particular time of day, or does it occur with exertion? Ask the patient if they have a cough. If so, is the cough productive(able to expel mucus), moist (sounds wet, but no mucus is expelled), or dry? Ask what color of sputum is produced, how often, and how much. Ask if there has been a change in the amount, color, or consistency of the mucus. It is not uncommon for a smoker to have a chronic cough, especially upon awakening. A cough can be a symptom of a common cold or a sign that the patient has significant disease, such as heart failure, emphysema, or lung cancer. An acute cough (related to a common cold) typically lasts for 3 weeks or less. A chronic cough has been present for more than 2 months. Increased mucus production or change in color can signify worsening of respiratory disease or other undiagnosed pathology. Ask the patient if there is any blood in the sputum (mucus). Hemoptysis (blood in the sputum) can signify lung cancer (blood-streaked sputum), tuberculosis (blood-streaked or bloody sputum), or heart failure (pink and frothy sputum). Ask the patient if they experience any wheezing. Wheezing is narrowing of the airways and can be caused by inflammation or presence of a foreign body.

Risk Factors Related to the System

An increased risk of developing respiratory disease exists in patients who smoke and those who are exposed to inhaled irritants. Smoking is the leading cause of preventable respiratory disease.

Risk Evaluation

Determine the amount of smoke exposure by calculating pack-years of smoking. Multiply the packs of cigarettes smoked per day times the number of years the patient smoked. (Packs per day) × (years of smoking) = pack-years. One pack-year is the equivalent of smoking one pack (20 cigarettes) per day for 1 year. It is important to determine the pack-years even if the patient no longer smokes. Exposure to tobacco smoke increases the risk of developing lung cancer or chronic obstructive pulmonary disease (COPD). An example of COPD is emphysema and chronic bronchitis.

Ask the patient about inhaled irritants, such as smoke (firefighters), coal dust (miners), flour dust (bakery workers), or industrial chemicals (such as toluene), to which they have been exposed. Ask about a history of exposure to asbestos. Exposure to asbestos increases the risk of developing mesothelioma.

ALERT

Patients who have chronic conditions or are at risk for respiratory disease should have an influenza vaccine (flu shot) every year. The vaccine is developed based on the anticipated strain or strains of influenza that are expected. Flu season in the USA typically occurs between December and March. The vaccine is recommended for women who will be pregnant during flu season. Therefore, the best time for vaccination is in early to mid-Fall.

Pneumococcal vaccine is recommended for those with chronic conditions, impaired immune systems, smokers, and those over the age of 65 years.

Objective Information

Equipment Needed

Stethoscope, pulse oximeter.

Assessment Techniques

Inspection, palpation, percussion, and auscultation.

Physical Examination

Inspection

Assess the patient's skin color and effort of respiration. Cyanosis occurs when there is not enough oxygen supply to the tissues that need it. The nail beds are also helpful in assessing oxygenation to the peripheral tissues. Check the mucus membranes if you are having difficulty with assessing the skin or nail beds. Cosmetics, tattoos, rashes, or nail polish can impair your ability to adequately assess color of the skin or nailbeds. Respirations should occur evenly and without undue effort. Note the rate and pattern of the respirations. Note the effort of respiration and if any accessory muscles are used. Muscle retractions between the ribs (intercostal retractions), above the clavicle (supraclavicular), and the presence of abdominal breathing in an adult are all signs that the patient is working harder than normal to breathe.

Patients resting comfortably are having an easy time with respiration. When patients are having difficulty breathing, they may sit upright and lean forward, resting their forearms on a table or back of a chair for support. This is referred to as a tripod position. Patients that are expending more energy to breathe may become diaphoretic (sweaty) from the effort.

Is the patient able to speak without difficulty? The more effort that is needed to breathe, the fewer words the patient can say without needing to take a breath. The fewer words between breaths, the more difficulty the patient is having.

Check peripheral oxygenation by using pulse oximetry. Oxygen is carried by (or attached to) hemoglobin and transported through the circulation. A pulse

TABLE 7-1 Normal Respiratory Rate Levels		
Stage	Age Range	Respiratory Rate, Breaths per Minute
Newborn	Birth to 3 mo	35-55
Infant	3-6 mo	30-45
	6-12 mo	25-40
Toddler	1-3 y	20-30
Preschooler	3-6 y	20-25
School-aged child	6-12 y	14-22
Adolescent and adult	Over 12 y	12-20

oximeter uses light-emitting diodes to calculate the percentage of hemoglobin that is carrying oxygen. It is most commonly used to detect the oxygenation levels by inserting a finger into the device. Normal pulse oximeter readings should be between 95 and 100. Readings below 90 indicate the need for supplemental oxygen. The pulse oximeter cannot distinguish between the presence of oxygen and carbon monoxide. Carbon monoxide can attach to the hemoglobin (displacing oxygen) and there may be a reading within normal range in patients with carbon monoxide exposure.

Palpation

Check for chest excursion and transmitted breath sounds by palpation.

Determine symmetry of chest expansion by placing your hands on the patient's back at the lower costal margins, with your thumbs toward the spine. Ask the patient to take a deep breath. Both hands should move laterally when the patient inhales and return to the initial position when they exhale.

Check for tenderness of the ribs or junction of the ribs, cartilage, and sternum by gently palpating the areas.

Mild vibration in noted along the chest wall when the patient speaks. This is called tactile fremitus. Assess both the right and the left sides of the chest simultaneously. Ask the patient to say 'ninety-nine' as you place your hands against the chest wall. Use the ulnar surface (pinky side) of your hand to assess the vibration. Systematically assess the entire posterior surface of the chest followed by the anterior surface.

Percussion

Percussion is typically assessed when the patient is sitting upright. There should be resonance on percussion of the air-filled lung. Place your index or middle finger from your nondominant hand within an intercostal space on the patient's chest wall. Quickly strike the distal interphalangeal joint (last knuckle) of your nondominant hand with the tip of your index (or middle) finger of your dominant hand. Avoid percussing over bony areas as this will result in a dull sound. Start at the top of the posterior chest, percussing on one side followed by the other and move systematically over the chest alternating from one side to the other until the entire chest is covered. Repeat on the anterior chest. The sound produced should be resonant, as if over an air-filled area.

Auscultation

Auscultation is typically performed with the patient sitting upright. Use the diaphragm of the stethoscope to listen to the anterior chest and then the posterior chest. Alternate from right to left and compare the sounds on each side. Ask the patient to take a deep breath and inhale and exhale through their mouth. Listen to a full respiratory cycle (inhalation and exhalation) at each location. Begin at the second intercostal space on the right near the sternal border (near the edge of the sternum) and then listen at the second intercostal space on the left near the sternal border. Move laterally on the left and then listen to the right side. Move down on the right side and then listen on the left. Continue to listen to one side, then the other until you have covered the entire anterior chest. When listening to the breath sounds of a female patient, you may need to gently displace the breast tissue to hear well. You may ask the patient to assist with this. The right middle lobe must be assessed either anteriorly or laterally between the fourth and sixth ribs.

The stethoscope should be placed directly upon the chest wall. Clothes may produce interference of the sounds. Remember to drape the patient's gown appropriately for modesty when assessing the chest.

TABLE 7-2		
	Breath Sound	**Location**
Tracheal	Higher pitch Inspiratory phase of respiration (I) = expiratory phase of respiration (E) very loud	Over the trachea—neck
Bronchial	Higher pitch I < E loud	Over the bronchus—upper sternum and on either side of the upper sternum
Broncho-vesicular	Intermediate pitch I = E intermediate	Over the larger airways—near sternal border or between shoulder blades
Vesicular	Lower pitch I > E soft	Over the smaller airways—most of the lung fields

Expected Findings

Respirations should be even and unlabored. The patient's color should have pink undertones. The respirations should be symmetrical, even, and unlabored. The width of the chest should be about twice that of the anterior–posterior diameter in an adult patient. There should not be any tenderness to palpation of the chest wall. There should be mild tactile fremitus. Percussion should reveal a resonant tone. Auscultation should reveal clear air exchange.

Abnormal Findings

Cyanosis may be seen if adequate oxygen is not reaching the tissues. Peripheral cyanosis occurs in the most distal areas—fingers, toes, tip of the nose. Central cyanosis occurs centrally (lips, face, trunk) and is more ominous.

Increased respiratory effort warrants further investigation. Use of accessory muscles denotes increased effort of breathing. Patients may have retractions of the intercostal, supraclavicular, or neck area. Mild use of abdominal muscles to aid respiration may be seen when patients are lying on their backs in bed as the posterior chest does not expand due to body weight. Abdominal breathing (using the abdominal muscles to aid chest expansion) is not normally seen in adults and signals increased respiratory effort when present.

Pectus excavatum: A sunken or concave appearance of the lower anterior chest.

Barrel chest: It is the term used when the anterior-posterior diameter increases. This is typically seen in COPD and is associated with hyperinflation of the lungs and a flattening of the diaphragm.

Tactile fremitus: Increased vibration is noted when palpating over an area of consolidation (such as pneumonia) while the patient is speaking. A decrease in the expected vibration may occur when there is an effusion (collection of fluid). Percussion over an area of consolidation will cause a dull sound.

Crackles (rales): A discontinuous bubbling or rattling sound which can be moist or dry, fine or coarse, produced by the presence of fluid in the airways.

Rhonchi: A continuous sound similar to snoring occurs when the airways are narrowed. The narrowing may be due to inflammation or the presence of mucus. If the patient coughs, the mucus may move and the location of the rhonchi will also move.

Wheezes: High-pitched continuous sounds that may occur in narrowed airways, more commonly on expiration.

Stridor: It is similar to a wheeze, created by obstruction in the major airway.

Bronchophony: Transmitted voice sounds that are clear and more easily understood over an area of consolidation.

Egophony: Transmitted voice sounds that produce an 'A' sound when the patient says 'E' that occur over an area of consolidation.

Whispered pectoriloquy: Transmitted whisper that is clear and more easily understood over an area of consolidation.

Age-Related Changes

Pediatric

Children have smaller airways and are more susceptible to problems with inflammation of the airways. The majority of pediatric cardiopulmonary arrests are due to respiratory causes. The cricoid cartilage that surrounds the trachea is smaller than the thyroid cartilage in small children. This creates an airway that is more funnel shaped than in the adult, where the airway has a more even diameter.

Use of the abdominal muscles during respiration (or abdominal breathing) is a normal finding in infants and small children.

Respiratory rate varies from the rapid rate of a newborn to the more adult-like rate of a school-aged child. Knowing the normal respiratory rate expected according to the age of the patient makes identification of abnormal findings easier.

Geriatric

There is a loss of elastic recoil within the lungs as people age. Lifetime exposure to inhaled irritants increases the possibility of respiratory disease later in life. Prevalence of COPD increases in the older population.

Cultural Considerations

There is not a great deal of cultural variation when it comes to breathing. Smoking is less common than it used to be, but is still accepted in certain groups. Certain occupations increase the risk of exposure to inhaled irritants.

Some people do not want to get vaccinated due to religious or other personal beliefs.

CASE STUDY

Jim is a 68-year-old retired construction worker who has a daily, moist, morning cough. He is an ex-smoker and has a history of occupational exposure to sawdust, asbestos, and other fine particulates. He has no other health problems.

REVIEW QUESTIONS

1. The normal expected respiratory rate for a 68-year-old patient is:
   A. 25-40.
   B. 20-30.
   C. 20-25.
   D. 12-20.

2. A daily, chronic cough is more common in:
   A. healthcare workers.
   B. smokers.
   C. athletes.
   D. teachers.

3. Due to a history of smoking, Jim would have an increased risk for the development of:
   A. chronic obstructive pulmonary disease (COPD).
   B. tuberculosis.
   C. pectus excavatum.
   D. tactile fremitus.

4. Rhonchi are adventitious breath sounds that are caused by:
   A. the presence of fluid in the airways.
   B. narrowing of the airways.
   C. percussing over an area of consolidation.
   D. obstruction of a large airway.

5. **The trachea bifurcates into the left and right main stem bronchus. This is located at approximately the level of the:**

    A. first thoracic vertebra.

    B. fourth to sixth intercostal space.

    C. Angle of Louis anteriorly and the fourth thoracic vertebrae posteriorly.

    D. xyphoid process.

6. **Which of the following occupations would increase the risk of a chronic respiratory disease?**

    A. Firefighter

    B. Coal miner

    C. Baker

    D. Construction worker

    E. All of the above

7. **Which ribs do not attach to the sternum or the cartilage of the ribs above?**

    A. 1 and 2

    B. 5 and 6

    C. 8 and 9

    D. 11 and 12

8. **When interviewing a newly hospitalized patient who is experiencing shortness of breath, you should:**

    A. use open-ended questions that encourage the patient to expand on their answers with details.

    B. use closed-ended questions that require short answers.

    C. complete the entire admission assessment as it is to be completed when the patient is first admitted.

    D. sit silently near the patient and wait for them to initiate conversation.

9. **Breathing is normally triggered by the respiratory drive. In an otherwise healthy individual, breathing is triggered by:**

    A. central chemoreceptors detecting an increase in carbon dioxide level ($PaCO_2$) within the arteries.

    B. peripheral chemoreceptors detecting a decrease in oxygen (PaO_2) levels.

    C. central chemoreceptors detecting an increase in carbon dioxide ($PaCO_2$) levels.

    D. peripheral chemoreceptors detecting an increase in oxygen (PaO_2) levels.

10. You are assessing Jim's oxygenation by using a pulse oximeter. You see a reading of 97%. You know that this is:

A. a sign of impending respiratory failure.

B. elevated.

C. within normal range.

D. decreased.

ANSWERS

1. D. 25-40 is the expected rate for a 6- to 12-month old infant.

   20-30 is the expected rate for a toddler.

   20-25 is the expected rate for a preschooler.

2. B. Healthcare workers, athletes, and teachers would not have a chronic cough.

3. A. Tuberculosis and pectus excavatum are not caused by smoking. Tactile fremitus is a normal finding.

4. B. Fluid in the airways produces fine crackles (rales). Rhonchi are auscultated, not percussed. Partial obstruction of a large airway results in stridor.

5. C. The right middle lobe is located between the fourth and sixth intercostal spaces. The right middle lobe is located anteriorly between the fourth and sixth rib area on the right side.

6. E. All of these occupations increase the risk for inhaled particulates, which increase the risk of developing chronic respiratory disease.

7. D. Ribs 1 through 7 attach directly to the sternum. Ribs 8 through 10 attach to the costal cartilage of the ribs above. Ribs 11 and 12 are free floating.

8. B. Questions with one-word or short answers are best when a patient is experiencing shortness of breath. Longer answers require more effort and will cause fatigue.

9. A. Central chemoreceptors detect an increase in carbon dioxide level ($PaCO2$) within the arteries and initiate respiration.

10. C. A normal pulse oximetry range is between 95%-100%

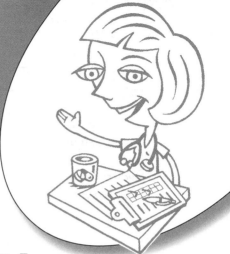

chapter **8**

Assessment of the Cardiovascular and Peripheral Vascular System

LEARNING OBJECTIVES

After reviewing this chapter, the learner will be able to:

1. Identify important anatomic landmarks of the cardiovascular system.
2. Discuss the appropriate information to gather during an interview.
3. Demonstrate a physical assessment of the cardiovascular system.
4. List normal physical assessment findings.
5. Describe abnormal physical assessment findings.
6. Discuss the age-related differences related to the cardiovascular system.

KEYWORDS

Atrioventricular node	Superior vena cava
Cardiac output	Syncope
Diastole	Systole
Mediastinum	Tricuspid valve
Stroke volume	Ventricular depolarization

Review of Anatomy and Physiology

The cardiovascular system contains the heart which is a muscular pump that beats an average of 60-100 times per minute in an adult, propelling blood into the lungs and then to the rest of the body. The heart is located in the mediastinum, an area in the middle of the chest containing the heart and the great vessels. The great vessels are the vena cava, pulmonary artery, pulmonary vein, and aorta (see Figure 8-1). The adult heart extends from the second rib to the fifth intercostal space with two-thirds of the heart mass lying left of the midsternal line. The heart is slightly rotated in the chest resulting in the anterior most aspect of the heart within the chest being the ventricles.

The outermost layer of the heart is the pericardium that consists of an outer fibrous layer and a thin inner layer. The inner layer is further divided into two layers: visceral and parietal. Between these two layers is about 30-50 milliliters (mL) of fluid that reduces friction when the heart contracts and relaxes. The myocardium is the muscular, middle layer of the heart consisting of striated cardiac muscle and performs the majority of the heart's work upon contraction. The innermost layer is the endocardium composed of smooth endothelial cells and lines the heart and the valves.

The heart is composed of four chambers: two top chambers called atria and two lower chambers called ventricles (see Figure 8-2). The septal wall separates the right and left sides of the heart. The right atrium receives unoxygenated blood from the body and right ventricle pumps it into the lungs. The left atrium receives oxygenated blood from the lungs and the left ventricle pumps the blood to the rest of the body. The heart has four valves to prevent the backflow of blood. In between the right atria and the right ventricle is the tricuspid valve which consists of three flaps that close upon atrial contraction, thereby preventing the flow of the deoxygenated blood (received from the body) back into the right atrium. On the left side of the body, the mitral valve, located in-between

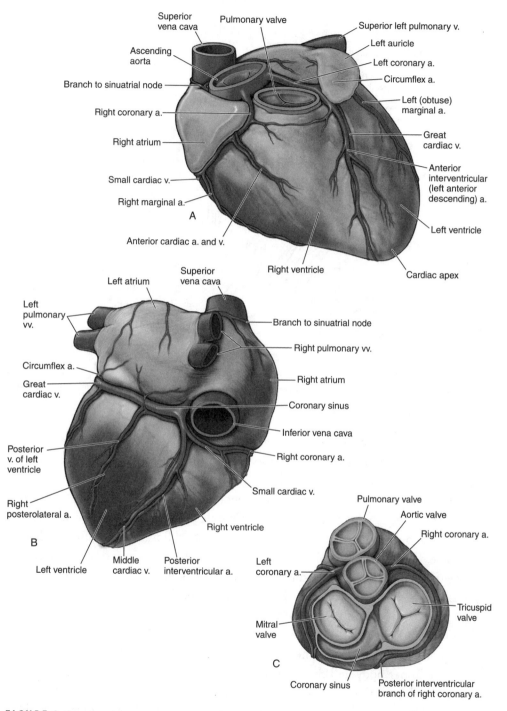

FIGURE 8-1 • Anatomy of the heart. Anterior (A), posterior (B), and superior (C) views. (Reproduced with permission from Morton DA, Foreman KB, Albertine KH: *The Big Picture: Gross Anatomy.* New York, NY: McGraw-Hill; 2011. Figure 4-2.)

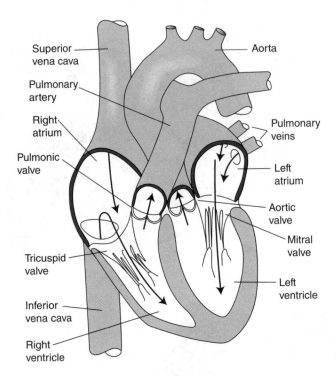

FIGURE 8-2 • Illustration of heart chambers showing direction of blood flow.
(Reproduced with permission from Mohrman DE, Heller LJ: *Cardiovascular Physiology*, 7th edition. New York, NY: McGraw-Hill; 2011. Figure 1-4.)

the left atrium and the left ventricle, prevents the backflow of oxygenated blood (received from the lungs) back into the left atrium. The tricuspid valve and the mitral valve are collectively called the atrioventricular (AV) valves (between the atria and the ventricles). The sound generated when the tricuspid valve and the mitral valve close is called S1. The pulmonic valve is located between right ventricle and the pulmonary artery and prevents backflow of blood into the left ventricle. The aortic valve is located between the left ventricle and the aorta and prevents the backflow of blood from the aorta back into the left ventricle. The pulmonic valve and the aortic valve are collectively called the semilunar (SL) valves (between the ventricles and the great vessels). The sound generated when the pulmonic valve and the aortic valve close is called S2.

Direction of blood flow: The superior vena cava returns blood to the heart from the upper body and the inferior vena cava returns blood from the lower body. Blood from the vena cava enters the right atrium, flows through the tricuspid valve and into the right ventricle. The deoxygenated blood flows through the pulmonary valve to the pulmonary artery (the only artery carrying unoxygenated blood) and then to the lungs. This oxygenated blood from the lungs enters the left atrium and flows through the mitral valve into the left ventricle. From the left ventricle, the blood flows through the aortic valve into the aorta and the rest of the body.

Cardiac cycle: A full cardiac cycle consists of diastole and systole. Diastole is the filling or resting state of the ventricles. During diastole the ventricles are relaxed and the tricuspid and mitral valves are open and blood is flowing freely into the ventricles. Most of the blood flowing into the ventricles occurs during the first third of diastole called the rapid filling period. Normally, there is no sound auscultated at this time in the undiseased heart. The atria contract and the last amount of blood enters the ventricles and the tricuspid and mitral valve snap shut. Atrial kick is the term used to define the force of atrial contraction pushing the last amount of blood into the ventricles. The sound generated from the closing of the tricuspid valve and the mitral valve is called S1. The closure of the AV valves producing the first heart sound begins systole. All valves are briefly closed. Pressure in the ventricles rises as the ventricles contract and causes the SL valves to open. This is now the ejection period and blood is ejected from the ventricles into the great vessels: the pulmonary artery on the right side of the heart and the aorta on the left side of the heart. The ejection fraction indicates the amount of blood ejected from the ventricles of the heart during systole. The average amount in a undiseased heart is 50%-70% of the total amount of the blood in the ventricles. As pressure falls at the end of systole the SL valves snap shut, and the sound generated when the pulmonic valve and the aortic valve close is called S2.

Electrical conduction of the heart: Cardiac muscle is distinctive from the other muscle cells in the body because it has the properties of automaticity and contractility. Automaticity is the ability to produce electric impulses that conduct through the heart. The electrical impulses generated are called action potentials that result in excitation of the muscle fibers all the way through the heart. The sinoatrial (SA) node, located in the right atrium initiates the electrical impulse. The SA node is considered the natural pacemaker of the heart. The impulse travels through the atria and continues to the AV node, located in the septal wall between the atria (interatrial septum). The AV junction located in the septal wall slows the conduction of the impulse as it connects the one-way conduction between the atria and the ventricles. The impulse is briefly delayed at the AV node allowing the atria to complete the ejection of blood before the impulse continues to the AV bundle. Once through the AV bundle the impulse travels to the right and left bundles of the Purkinje system, which causes the ventricles to contract together.

The SA node starts the impulse with a steady rhythm of 60-100 beats per minute in an adult. If the SA node fails to start the impulse, then the AV node can initiate an impulse at a rate of 40-60 beats per minute. The Purkinje fibers can also generate an impulse of 15-40 beats per minute. The AV node and the Purkinje fibers do not normally generate an impulse because the SA node discharges at a faster rate and only "take over" if the SA node fails to function.

The electrocardiogram (ECG) is a test that reveals the recording of the electrical activity of the heart. Each beat of the heart is shown as a wave on a chart recorder with deflection points designated for atrial depolarization (P wave), ventricular depolarization (QRS wave), and ventricular repolarization (T wave) (see Figure 8-3). Atrial depolarization is the conduction of the impulse throughout the atria and atrial repolarization, the relaxation of the atria is hidden in the QRS wave and is therefore not visible. Ventricular depolarization is the conduction of the impulse throughout the ventricles and ventricular repolarization is the relaxation of the ventricles.

Cardiac output: The amount of blood the heart pumps each minute is termed cardiac output (CO), which measures how well the heart is working as a pump. The CO is defined by the stroke volume (SV), the amount of blood pumped out of the left ventricle in one beat or contraction, multiplied by the

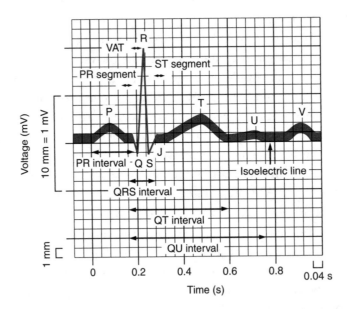

FIGURE 8-3 • Sample of ECG graph.
P: atrial depolarization; PR interval: the start of atrial depolarization to the start of ventricular depolarization; QRS: ventricular depolarization; ST segment: ventricular depolarization to the beginning of ventricular repolarization; T: ventricular repolarization; QT: interval – time for ventricular depolarization + ventricular repolarization; U wave: final phase of ventricular repolarization.
(Reproduced with permission from Gomella LG, Haist SA: *Clinician's Pocket Reference*, 11th edition. New York, NY: McGraw-Hill; 2007. Figure 19-2.)

heart rate (HR), the number of times the heart beats in 1 minute. The normal range of beats per minute is 60-100 beats in an adult. The CO varies with exercise, rest, and the metabolic needs of the body. It increases with exercise and decreases with rest or sleep. The CO is measured by liters per minute (L/min) with the average adult pumping 5 L/min.

EXAMPLE:

Miss Jones has an HR of 72 beats per minute and an SV of 70 mL/beat. What is her cardiac output (CO)?

$$CO = HR \times SV$$
$$CO = 72 \text{ (beats per minute)} \times 70 \text{ (mL/beat)} = 5040 \text{ mL/min.}$$

The CO is dependent on the amount of blood that is returning to the heart. Preload is the amount of stretch that the returning blood exerts on the muscle fibers of the heart at the end of diastole, the greater the stretch the greater the contraction of the heart. Afterload is the work the heart must produce to push the blood from the left ventricle into the aorta. Systemic arterial blood pressure, the pulmonary arterial pressure, atherosclerosis, and stenosis of the aortic valve and the pulmonic valve will determine the amount of work the heart must produce in order to push the blood into the aorta and the pulmonary artery.

The arterial system of the peripheral vascular system consists of arteries, which are thick-walled vessels that are elastic so that they can expand and relax to allow blood flow, and arterioles, which consist of one or two layers of smooth muscle to regulate the flow of blood into the capillaries. The capillaries connect the arterial system with the venous system and are one cell in thickness. The venules are thin walled and collect the blood from the capillaries and direct the blood into the veins that have a series of valves to prevent the backflow of blood. Venous blood is moved toward the heart by the muscular contractions.

A careful review of the peripheral vascular system includes assessing the pulses found throughout the body. A pulse can be found when a superficial artery is compressed against an underlying bone as a rush of blood flows through the artery.

> ## ALERT
>
> Where to palpate the arterial pulses of the body:
>
> **Temporal artery:** In the temple area, anterior to the natural hair-line by top of the ear.
>
> **Carotid artery:** In the space between the sternomastoid muscle and the trachea.
>
> **Arm:** Brachial, radial, ulnar
>
>   **Brachial:** About 0.5 inch above the antecubital fossa of the elbow, on the medial side.
>
>   **Radial:** Medial to the radius bone on dorsal side of the hand upward, proximal to the thumb.
>
>   **Ulnar:** Medial on the wrist with the palm turned upward.
>
> **Leg:** Femoral, popliteal, posterior tibial, dorsalis pedis
>
>   **Femoral:** Under the inguinal ligament in the groin area.
>
>   **Popliteal:** In the midarea, behind the patella or kneecap.
>
>   **Posterior tibial:** Below the medial malleolus in the groove between the medial malleolus and the Achilles tendon.
>
>   **Dorsalis pedis:** Dorsum of the foot; below, proximal to and parallel to the great toe.
>
> **Heart:** Apical
>
>   **Apical:** Between the fourth and fifth intercostal space, to the left side, midclavicular line in an adult.

Subjective Information

Interview

The interview of a patient to assess for cardiac disease needs to be quick and efficient if he/she is currently experiencing chest pain. If the patient is new to the healthcare provider and is currently not experiencing chest pain, then the following review of systems (ROS) questions can be asked.

Review of Systems

Ask the patient about any episodes of pain or discomfort in the chest, neck, jaw, or upper back. Have you experienced chest, jaw, or upper back pain? If pain is present or has occurred, ask the patient if they can point to the area. Have the patient describe the quality of the pain (sharp, dull, tightness, stabbing, burning, etc). Ask about the duration of the pain. Does it last for seconds, minutes, or longer? Ask about any radiation of the pain to other areas. For example, the pain may begin on the anterior chest in the area of the third and fourth intercostal space at the sternal border and radiate to the left jaw. Determine if the pain occurs with exertion, at rest, or both. Have the patient rate the pain on a scale of 1-10, with 1 being mild and 10 being the worst pain imagined. Ask if the pain resolves with rest or if medication, such as nitroglycerin, is needed. Ask about the presence of any associated symptoms, such as palpitations, shortness of breath, excessive sweating, nausea, vomiting, lightheadedness, or dizziness. Can you point to the area where the pain occurs? How long does the pain last? Does the pain radiate anywhere, for example: down your left arm or to the upper back or jaw? Can you describe the pain, for example: stabbing, tightness, burning, throbbing, sharp, or dull pain? Do you have any symptoms with the pain, for example: nausea, vomiting, shortness of breath, palpitations, or excessive sweating? Does the pain go away with rest or do you take medication, for example: sublingual nitroglycerin? Angina, acute coronary syndrome, or myocardial infarction cause chest discomfort. It is important to quickly determine as much information as possible about the pain or discomfort that the patient is experiencing. There may also be noncardiac causes for substernal or epigastric area pain. Heartburn, gallbladder disease, gastric ulcer, or respiratory disorders may also cause discomfort that is similar in location to cardiac causes.

Associated Symptoms

1. **Dyspnea**–Do you have any difficulty with breathing or have labored breathing? Is it on exertion or at rest? Dyspnea on exertion may signal congestive heart failure. Does the shortness of breath wake you up at night? Paroxysmal nocturnal dyspnea (PND) occurs when the patient wakes up suddenly after being asleep for 2-4 hours and feels shortness of breath and needs to sit or stand to relieve the shortness of breath.
2. **Fatigue**–Do you experience fatigue when performing your normal daily activities? Does anyone in your family complain that you are getting "lazy?"
3. **Cough**–Do you experience a cough? When does the cough occur? Is the cough a dry cough or does it bring up sputum? If yes, what is the color of the sputum and can you estimate the amount? Does the cough occur at night after you have been sleeping? How many pillows do you use while sleeping?
4. **Syncope**–Have you ever "blacked out" or experienced dizziness? Do you feel dizzy when you sit up or stand up suddenly?

5. **Retention of fluid**–Do your ankles swell? If yes, what time of the day do they swell? Have you gained any weight recently? Do you feel your shoes getting tighter? Do you need to get up at night to urinate?

6. **Heartburn**–Do you experience heartburn or burning under the sternal area or in your chest? Do you get chest pain after a large meal?

Risk Factors Related to the System

Coronary artery disease (CAD) is the most common type of heart disease and can lead to myocardial infarction (heart attack). Obesity and physical inactivity are the two major risk factors for the development of CAD, and the development of atherosclerosis starts in childhood. Patients at risk have a body mass index (BMI) over 25. BMI is determined by the patient's height and weight and correlates with the amount of body fat. Patients with high blood pressure, which injures the lining of the arteries, as well as high cholesterol and high triglyceride levels are at an increased risk of heart disease. Cigarette smoking has been clearly indicated in the development of heart disease, because smoking increases blood pressure, decreases exercise tolerance, and increases the tendency of the blood to clot. Patients with diabetes also have an increased risk of heart disease because of insulin resistance, high levels of triglycerides, and low levels of high-density lipoproteins (HDLs) that carry cholesterol back to the liver. It is important for the patients to know their family history of heart disease so that they can modify their other risk factors.

Atheromas (fatty deposits) develop in the intimal wall of the coronary arteries. This happens in a progressive fashion with the process beginning with endothelial injury and a focal deposit of cholesterol and lipids. A complicated lesion consists of plaque that contains a core of lipid materials within an area of dead tissue. With the incorporation of lipids, thrombi, damaged tissue, and accumulation of calcium, the growing lesion becomes complex and eventually completely blocks the flow of blood through the coronary arteries which leads to a myocardial infarction. The ischemic area ceases to function within minutes and irreversible damage (necrosis and death of cardiac tissue) can occur in 20-40 minutes. Chest pain is the classic symptom of a myocardial infarction that is not relieved with position change, rest, or sublingual nitrate administration.

Risk Evaluation

1. **Family history**–Does anyone in your family have a history of chest pain, hypertension, elevated cholesterol levels, or sudden death due to a heart attack (myocardial infarction)? At what age did the relative develop these

symptoms and are they a first-degree relative (mother, father, siblings)? A genogram compiled with the patient will show the patient's risk of heart disease by revealing the number of relatives with heart disease.

2. **Personal history**–Do you have a history of hypertension, high cholesterol or high triglycerides, congenital heart disease, chronic obstructive pulmonary disease (COPD), CAD, diabetes, or gastroesophageal reflux disease (GERD)? Many diseases of the respiratory system or gastrointestinal system have similar symptoms to cardiac disease.

3. **Personal habits**–Do you smoke cigarettes or marijuana? If yes, how many cigarettes a day do you smoke and how many years have you been smoking? (To determine pack-years, multiply the number of packs smoked daily with the number of years the patient has smoked.)
   Example: Miss Smith smoked two packs of cigarettes a day for 20 years.

$$2 \times 20 = 40 \text{ pack-years.}$$

If the patient stated that they smoked in the past, ask how old they were when they started smoking and when they quit, determining the number of years the patient smoked.

Self-Care Behaviors

Patients should quit smoking and eat a low-fat diet. Patients with a BMI over 25 should be counseled to lose weight and referred to a dietician. Advice on quitting smoking should be given to the patient upon each visit. Thirty minutes of moderate aerobic exercise is recommended daily. The patient's cholesterol levels should be checked including total cholesterol, HDL, low-density lipoprotein (LDL), and LDL particles. Patients with high cholesterol levels should be counseled concerning a low-fat diet and referred to a healthcare provider for lipid-lowering medication.

Objective Information

Equipment Needed

Stethoscope with a bell and a diaphragm, good lighting, two small centimeter rulers.

Assessment Techniques

Inspection, palpation, auscultation.

Physical Examination

Inspection of the Anterior Chest

With the patient in a supine position and the head of the bed at 30 degrees, inspect the anterior chest for pulsations or lifting of the chest wall.

Palpation of the Anterior Chest

Using the palmar aspect of the hand palpate across the anterior chest at the apex and base area of the heart as well as the left sternal border. Using the finger pads of your hand palpate the apical impulse at the midclavicular line between the fourth or fifth intercostal space on the patient's left side of the anterior chest. The patient may need to turn on his/her left side to assist the healthcare provider in finding the apical impulse.

Auscultation of the Anterior Chest for Heart Sounds

With the patient in a supine position and lying at a 30 degree angle, the healthcare provider should start listening at the apex of the heart for the rate and rhythm of the heart. If the room is noisy, eliminate all noise by turning off the TV and closing the door of the room. Have the patient breathe normally. The healthcare provider can further put his/her chin down and close the eyes and concentrate on the sounds generated by the heart. The healthcare provider should practice listening to several undiseased hearts to gain an understanding of the normal sounds generated by the heart. Listen to the heart for a full minute to assess the rate and rhythm of the heart. Identification of S1 (lub) is performed by listening at the apex of the heart and S1 correlates with the carotid pulse, and identification of S2 (dub) is performed at the base of the heart and directly follows S1.

ALERT

The healthcare provider should further auscultate the anterior chest at the four areas where the valves of the heart radiate as follows:

1. Aortic area: Second intercostal space to the right of the sternum.
2. Pulmonic area: Second intercostal space to the left of the sternum.
3. Tricuspid area: Left sternal border at the fourth or fifth intercostal space.

> 4. Mitral area: Apex of the heart at the fourth or fifth intercostal space, midclavicular line.
>
> First, listen at each area with the diaphragm and then the bell of the stethoscope.

Expected Findings of Palpation of the Peripheral Arteries

Inspection of the Anterior Chest

There should be no pulsations or lifting of the chest wall.

Palpation of the Anterior Chest

There should be no pulsations of the chest wall. The apical impulse is about 1×2 cm in width and is normally a short tap on the healthcare provider's finger pads. The apical impulse will be difficult to assess in an obese patient and in a patient with large breasts.

Auscultation of the Anterior Chest for Heart Sounds

The normal rate of the adult heart is between 60 and 100 beats per minute and the normal rhythm is regular. Two sounds are normally generated by the heart: S1 coincides with the closing of the tricuspid and mitral valves; and S2 coincides with the closing of the pulmonic and aortic valves. Auscultation at each of the four areas where the valves radiate sound reveal no extra sounds or murmurs. A split S2 can be heard by the trained ear with inspiration as the aortic valve closes before the pulmonic valve and is heard as a beat at the pulmonic area (second-left intercostal space).

Abnormal Findings

Inspection of the Anterior Chest

A lifting or pulsation on the chest wall may reveal an enlarged heart that is working hard to move blood through the ventricles.

Palpation of the Anterior Chest

A palpable vibration is called a thrill and reveals turbulent blood flow through the heart. A displaced apical impulse toward the left axilla could possibly reveal an enlarged left ventricle (left ventricle hypertrophy).

Auscultation of the Anterior Chest for Heart Sounds

An HR slower than 60 beats per minute is called bradycardia and an HR faster than 100 beats per minute is called tachycardia. A rate that is bradycardic or tachycardic can affect the CO of the heart. An irregular rhythm can be caused by an arrhythmia of the heart and further investigation of the cause is necessary.

An extra sound or murmur heard at one of the four areas where the valves radiate sound might indicate an abnormality of the corresponding valve.

Extra Heart Sounds

S3 and S4 are sounds generated from blood entering a noncompliant ventricle. They are heard best at the apex of the heart with the bell of the stethoscope. These sounds usually indicate fluid overload and are seen in patients with a history of coronary heart disease, congestive heart failure, ischemic heart disease, and other heart conditions.

Murmurs

The healthcare provider should auscultate for a swishing sound across the entire precordium with the diaphragm and then the bell of the stethoscope. Murmurs are heard when there is turbulent blood flow within the heart. Auscultate first with the patient in the supine position with the head of the bed at 30 degrees, then with the patient in the left lateral position, and then with the patient sitting up and leaning forward. A positive murmur in any of these positions could indicate: backflow of blood (regurgitation) or obstruction of flow through a valve that has a narrow opening (stenosis).

TABLE 8-1   Grading of Heart Murmurs
Grade 1: Barely heard.
Grade 2: Soft sound, but easily heard.
Grade 3: Moderately loud.
Grade 4: Loud with a palpable thrill.
Grade 5: Very loud with a palpable thrill.
Grade 6: Heard without the stethoscope on the chest.

ALERT

If the healthcare provider auscultates a murmur, it should be documented as follows:

- The position the patient was in when the murmur was heard.
- The area on the chest where the murmur was the most prominent.
- The type of sound generated by the murmur: intensity, pitch.
- If the sound radiated to another area of the chest.
- If the sound changed, when the patient changed position.
- Grade of murmur.

This information would be documented along with the subjective complaints offered by the patient as well as a cardiac health history.

Age-Related Changes

Pediatric

Children can be born with a variety of heart conditions, and assessment of the child or infant is of the utmost importance. Vital signs including an apical HR could alert to cardiac problems. It is essential to note respiratory changes with a rapid HR (tachycardia) that could indicate early heart failure. A sinus arrhythmia is considered normal, whereby the HR increases with inspiration and decreases with expiration. A splitting of S2 is heard easily a few hours after birth. Innocent murmurs are commonly heard in children without cardiac disease. However, the absence of a murmur does not rule out a cardiac condition and frequent observation and auscultation of the infant should be performed. Inspection begins with the mucous membranes, and central cyanosis is exhibited by a bluish tone around the mouth. Inspection of the nail beds for clubbing in children reveals long-standing oxygen deprivation of the peripheral tissues. Palpation of the infant and child's skin should be dry and extremities equally warm to touch. Capillary refill should be less than 3 seconds and is best assessed in the great toe in children. Auscultation of the lungs and heart can be performed simultaneously when the infant or child is quiet and can be performed when the child is sitting in the caretaker's lap.

Geriatric

A complaint of dizziness upon arising from a supine position to a sitting or standing position is termed orthostatic hypotension and can be assessed in the older adult. Auscultation of the blood pressure may also reveal a rise in the systolic blood pressure. The apical impulse may be difficult to assess in the geriatric patient with COPD due to the increased diameter of the anteroposterior diameter of the chest. If a missed or ectopic beat is palpated or auscultated with the apical pulse, the healthcare provider should obtain an ECG. The elderly patient's HR should not change as the patient ages.

Cultural Considerations

Heart disease remains the leading cause of death in the USA among all ethnicities for adults aged 65 years and older. Men of African descent are more likely to have poorly controlled hypertension and are commonly diagnosed at a later date than Caucasians or Hispanics. African American men are 30% more likely to die from heart disease than Caucasian men. Although Hispanics are 10% less likely to die from heart disease than non-Hispanic Caucasians, Mexican American women are 20% more likely to have hypertension than non-Hispanic Caucasian women and are more likely to suffer from obesity (CDC, 2010*). American Indian and Alaska native adults also have higher hypertension rates than Caucasians. Asian- Pacific Islanders are less likely to die from heart disease than Caucasians.

CASE STUDY

Mr Jones is a 56-year-old African American man with a history of hypertension. The healthcare provider is interviewing him today at the clinic. Mr Jones states that he "ran" out of his BP medication two weeks ago and does not have the money to buy his medication until the end of the month after he pays his rent and other bills. On assessment his BP is 180/90 mm Hg, Pulse 92, Respirations 24, and BMI 32. Mr Jones smokes one pack of cigarettes a day for 30 years and drinks 3-4 beers on the weekend.

---

*http://www.cdc.gov/nchs/data/databriefs/db48.pdf

REVIEW QUESTIONS

1. **The valve that is located between the right atrium and the right ventricle is called the:**
   A. mitral valve.
   B. tricuspid valve.
   C. pulmonic valve.
   D. aortic valve.

2. **The healthcare provider is auscultating Mr Jones' heart and hears lub dub (S1 and S2, respectively). S1 is best heard:**
   A. at the second right intercostal space.
   B. at the second left intercostal space.
   C. at the base of the heart.
   D. at the apex of the heart.

3. **The healthcare provider is auscultating the heart of a patient with coronary heart disease. If the heart rate (HR) is between 40 and 60 beats per minute, what part of the electrical conduction system might be initiating the heartbeat of the patient?**
   A. Sinoatrial (SA) node
   B. Atrioventricular (AV) node
   C. Purkinje fibers
   D. Bundle of His

4. **What risk factors does Mr Jones have for cardiac disease?** *Select all that apply.*
   A. Smoking
   B. Hypertension
   C. Ethnicity
   D. Gender

5. **The healthcare provider is auscultating Mr Jones' heart and notes an S3. What does the sound of an S3 indicate?**
   A. Turbulent blood flow.
   B. Stenosis of a valve.
   C. Regurgitation of blood flow.
   D. Noncompliant ventricle.

6. **What is Mr Jones' pack-years of smoking cigarettes?**
   A. 30 pack-years
   B. 60 pack-years
   C. 45 pack-years
   D. 15 pack-years

7. **What additional information would the healthcare provider need to further complete a heath history for Mr Jones?**

   A. Do you have a history of cancer?

   B. Does your mother or father have a history of heart disease?

   C. Have you applied for assistance to pay for your medication?

   D. Have you lost weight recently?

8. **The healthcare provider understands that a patient with a murmur with a palpable thrill is which of the following grades of murmurs?** *Select all that apply.*

   A. Grade II

   B. Grade III

   C. Grade IV

   D. Grade V

9. **The healthcare provider is palpating Mr Jones' apical impulse and finds it displaced laterally from the left midclavicular line. What does the he/she suspect?**

   A. Pleural effusion.

   B. Left ventricular hypertrophy.

   C. Pulmonic stenosis.

   D. Myocardial infarction.

10. **The P wave on the electrocardiogram (ECG) indicates:**

    A. atrial depolarization.

    B. ventricular repolarization.

    C. ventricular depolarization.

    D. atrial repolarization.

ANSWERS

1. B. The tricuspid is one of the atrioventricular (AV) valves and is located between the right atrium and the right ventricle.

2. D. S1 is best heard at the apex of the heart and S2 is best heard at the base of the heart.

3. B. The SA node produces an impulse at a rate of 60-100 beats per minute. The Purkinje fibers produce a rate of 15-40 beats per minute and the AV node produces a rate of 40-60 beats per minute, and the AV node and the Purkinje fibers only "take over" for the SA node when it fails to produce an impulse.

4. All of the above.

5. D. A murmur is commonly heard with turbulent blood flow and may or may not accompany an S3 sound. Stenosis of a valve is caused by a narrowed valve and can

cause a murmur, and regurgitation is backflow of blood and usually produces a murmur. S3 and S4 are sounds generated from blood entering a noncompliant ventricle.

6. A. $1 \times 30 = 30$ pack-years.

7. B. Having a first-degree relative with heart disease puts the patient at a higher risk for having heart disease.

8. B and C. A Grade IV and Grade V murmur would have a palpable thrill.

9. B. A displaced apical impulse could indicate an enlarged left ventricle (left ventricular hypertrophy).

10. A. The P wave indicates atrial depolarization (atrial contraction). The QRS indicates ventricular depolarization (ventricular contraction) and the T wave indicates ventricular repolarization (ventricular relaxation). Atrial repolarization (atrial relaxation) is buried in the QRS wave.

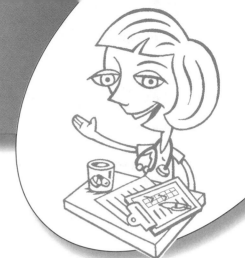

chapter 9

Assessment of the Abdomen, Pelvis, Anus, and Rectum

After reviewing this chapter, the learner will be able to:

❶ Identify important anatomic landmarks of the abdomen, pelvis, and rectum.

❷ Discuss the appropriate information to gather during an interview.

❸ Demonstrate a physical assessment of the abdomen, pelvis, and rectum.

❹ List normal physical assessment findings.

❺ Describe abnormal physical assessment findings.

❻ Discuss the age-related differences related to the abdomen, pelvis, and rectum.

KEYWORDS

Body mass index (BMI)
Calcitriol
Costovertebral angle (CVA)
Dysphagia
Fluid wave

Midclavicular line
Parietal peritoneum
Pyloric sphincter
Rebound tenderness
Viscera

Introduction

Assessment of the abdomen involves several different body systems. The gastrointestinal and genitourinary systems comprise the majority of the contents within the abdomen. Female reproductive organs are also located in the pelvic area. It is helpful to try to picture the underlying structures when performing the assessment.

Review of Anatomy and Physiology

The abdominal cavity extends from the xiphoid process of the sternum to the symphysis pubis, posteriorly by the vertebral column, and is bordered laterally by the abdominal muscles (see Figure 9-1). The internal abdominal cavity is lined with a thin protective membrane called the parietal peritoneum. The internal organs of the abdomen are called the viscera and consist of the solid viscera, which maintain a characteristic shape: for example, liver, spleen, pancreas, kidneys, ovaries, uterus, and adrenal glands, and the hollow viscera, which change shape based on contents inside: for example, bladder, gallbladder, stomach, small intestine, and colon.

The abdomen is divided into four quadrants for assessment: the right upper quadrant (RUQ), right lower quadrant (RLQ), left upper quadrant (LUQ), and left lower quadrant (LLQ) (see Figure 9-2). The abdomen can also be divided into nine sections: the right subcostal (below the ribs); right lumbar (the lateral middle area); right inguinal (from the anterior iliac crest to the inguinal area); the epigastric area (below the xiphoid process); the umbilical area (surrounding the umbilicus); the hypogastric or suprapubic area (above the symphysis pubis); the left subcostal (below the ribs); the left lumbar (the lateral middle area); and the left inguinal (from the anterior iliac crest to the inguinal area).

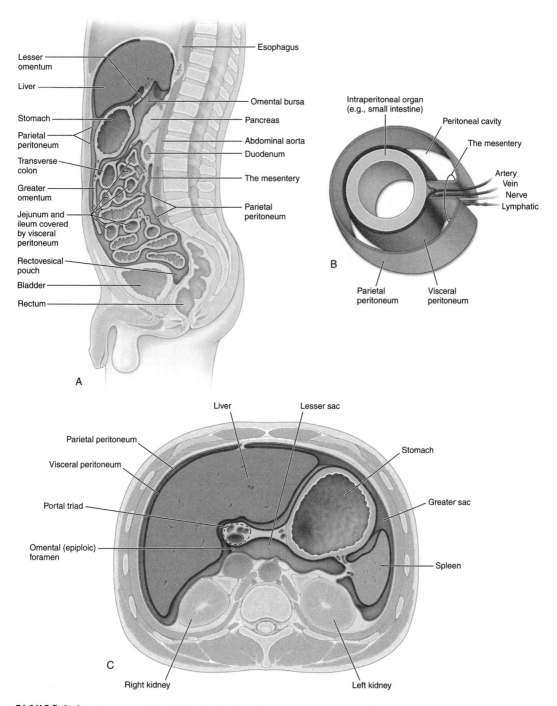

FIGURE 9-1 • Anatomy of the abdominal cavity.
(Reproduced with permission from Morton DA, Foreman KB, Albertine KH: *The Big Picture: Gross Anatomy*. New York, NY: McGraw-Hill; 2011. Figure 8-1.)

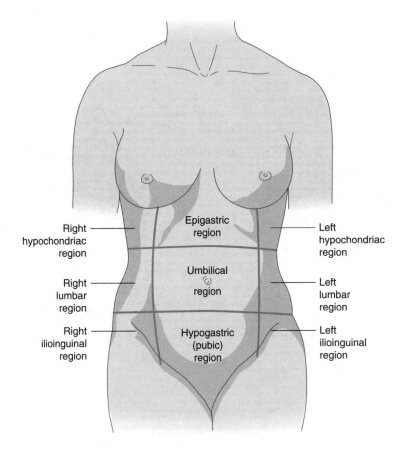

FIGURE 9-2 • Regions of the abdomen.
(Reproduced with permission from DeCherney AH, Nathan L, Laufer N et al: *Current Diagnosis & Treatment: Obstetrics & Gynecology*, 11th edition. New York, NY: McGraw-Hill; 2012. Figure 1-1.)

It is important to be aware of the structures in each area.

Structure and Function of Main Organs

Liver

Largest solid organ in the body, largely protected by the lower ribcage and located below the diaphragm in the RUQ extending to the left midclavicular line; metabolizes medications (or drugs); detoxifies substances; produces bile; stores fat-soluble vitamins, such as Vitamins A, D, and K; converts glucose to glycogen for storage, metabolizes proteins, carbohydrates, and fats; produces clotting factors and immune factors; excretes bilirubin; synthesizes, stores, and excretes cholesterol.

RUQ	LUQ
Liver	Stomach
Gallbladder	Spleen
Duodenum	Pancreatic body and tail
Ascending colon	Left kidney
Hepatic flexure of colon	Left adrenal gland
Transverse colon	Left ureter
Pancreatic head	Splenic flexure of colon
Right kidney	Transverse colon
Right adrenal gland	Descending colon
Right ureter	Uterus
Aorta	Aorta
Renal artery	Renal artery
RLQ	**LLQ**
Appendix	Left ovary
Cecum	Left fallopian tube
Ascending colon	Uterus
Right ovary	Left spermatic cord
Right fallopian tube	Left ureter
Uterus	Descending colon
Bladder	Sigmoid colon
Right ureter	Aorta
Right spermatic cord	Iliac artery
Aorta	
Iliac artery	

Gallbladder

Located beneath the liver, stores bile.

Pancreas

Extends from RUQ to LUQ; secretes digestive enzymes to aid in the breakdown of proteins, carbohydrates, and fats; secretes insulin to stimulate cells to use glucose (lowers blood glucose level); secretes glucagon, which raises the blood sugar level.

Spleen

Located in LUQ below the diaphragm at the level of 9th to 11th rib above the left kidney. It functions to remove old red blood cells and produces and stores white blood cells and platelets.

Kidneys

Located posteriorly in the upper abdomen, just below the diaphragm muscle, with the right kidney lower than the left because of the position of the liver. It functions to filter and remove metabolic waste products, helps to control blood pressure, and helps to maintain protein, fluid, and electrolyte balance. The nephrons within the kidney are comprised of intertwined glomerulus (capillaries which filter excess fluid and waste) and tubules (small tubes to collect urine). The kidneys release renin (aids in blood pressure control), erythropoietin (stimulates formation of red blood cells), and calcitriol (maintains calcium for use by bones, maintains electrolyte balance).

Stomach

Located in LUQ and functions to store and digest food by the secretion of necessary enzymes and by churning motions. The lower esophageal sphincter located between the esophagus and the stomach controls the movement of food and/or fluids between the esophagus and the stomach. The pyloric sphincter is located between the stomach and the small intestine and controls the movement of food and/or fluids from the stomach.

Small Intestine

Longest part of intestine is the small intestine and it is about 20-feet long. It is a hollow muscular tube and has three areas, duodenum, jejunum, and ileum, and is coiled in all four quadrants. Its main function is to further digest food and absorb nutrients.

Large Intestine or Colon

Starts in RLQ and terminates in the LLQ forming the sigmoid colon. The ascending colon extends along the right side of the abdomen; the transverse colon goes along the upper abdomen and descending colon extends along the left side of the abdomen. Water is absorbed throughout the large intestine.

Rectum

Lowest portion of large intestine and stores fecal material. Nerves within the rectum will signal the need to defecate.

Anal Canal

Final segment of digestive system ending at the anal opening, which is composed of an internal sphincter made of smooth, involuntary muscle and the external sphincter made of skeletal voluntary muscle.

Bladder

Located midline in the suprapubic area, but can extend to umbilicus when distended. Functions to store urine.

Subjective Information

Interview

The interview of the patient for the abdominal system concentrates on nutritional choices as well as specific questions about appetite, bowel habits, food intolerance, and food allergies. It is important to remember to ask questions about the patient's history, present concerns, family history and lifestyle, and complaints of abdominal pain.

Review of Systems (ROS)

Ask the patient specific questions about nutrition. What do you eat in a typical day? Performing a 24-hour nutritional recall will give insight about the foods commonly eaten. Has there been any change in your appetite or weight? Do you have any trouble swallowing food or liquids (dysphagia)? Trouble swallowing can indicate neuromuscular problems affecting the throat or esophagus. Do you experience discomfort before or after eating (indigestion)? The timing of heartburn or indigestion can help to determine the likely cause. Are there any foods that you cannot eat due to intolerance or food allergies? Also ask about the type of reaction that occurs.

Do you experience abdominal pain? If yes, ask the patient the following questions one at a time: Can you describe the pain (eg, is it cramping, sharp, or dull)? Can you point to the pain? Does it radiate anywhere? What is the characteristic of the pain? When does it occur (is it before or after meals)? and what, if anything, relieves the pain or makes it worse?

Have you been diagnosed with an abdominal condition? How often do you have a bowel movement? Describe the bowel movement. Has there been a recent change in your bowel movements? Recent changes in bowel movements (frequency, color, odor, diameter of stool may indicate significant pathology. Do you use laxatives or antacids? How often? Do you have any rectal bleeding or itching? Do you have any history of abdominal conditions or abdominal surgery? Are you taking any medication or over-the-counter (OTC) products, supplements, or herbal preparations?

Associated Symptoms

1. **Nausea**- Do you experience nausea? If yes, when do you experience it, before or after meals?
2. **Vomiting**- Do you have a history of vomiting? Is it intentional? What does the vomitus look like?
3. **Diarrhea**- Do you experience diarrhea? How often? Does it interfere with your lifestyle?
4. **Constipation**- Do you have a bowel movement(BM) less than every 3 days?(A patient should have a BM at least once every three days or more often) If yes, does a laxative relieve it? Do you eat a diet high in fiber and drink at least eight glasses of water a day?

ALERT

Body mass index (BMI) is an easy screening for the patient's risk of health problems related to being either overweight or underweight. In most cases, a simple chart (with height on one axis and weight on the other axis) will estimate the patient's BMI. It can be calculated by multiplying the weight in pounds over the height in inches squared by 703; or dividing the weight in kilograms by the height in meters squared.

$$\text{(Weight in pounds/height in inches squared)} \times 703 = \text{BMI}$$
$$\text{Weight in kilograms/height in meters squared} = \text{BMI}$$

BMI TABLE	
Underweight	18.5 or less
Normal weight	18.5–24.9
Overweight	25–29.9
Obese	30 or above

Risk Factors Related to the System

Patients with changes in appetite are at risk for electrolyte imbalances and anemia. Changes in appetite can indicate physiologic or psychologic disease. Unintentional weight loss can signal serious pathology. Daily use of laxatives may interfere with the body's natural ability to defecate when the laxatives are stopped. Frequent use of OTC antacids may result in electrolyte disturbances.

Risk Evaluation

1. **Family history**–Does anyone in your family have a history of an abdominal condition, for example, irritable bowel syndrome, ulcerative colitis, diverticulitis, or Crohn disease? If yes, at what age did it develop? How was this diagnosed and how is it being treated? What treatments have been successful?

2. **Personal history**–Do you have a personal history of nausea, vomiting, diarrhea, indigestion, or constipation? Do you have a history of any abdominal conditions, for example, ulcers, gastroesophageal reflux disease (GERD), gallbladder disease, hepatitis or liver disease? How was it diagnosed and how is it treated? Do you currently take any medications for the condition? If yes, do they successfully relieve symptoms? Have you ever had abdominal surgery? If so, what type of surgery? Do you have any current symptoms related to the surgery?

    What medications are you taking and do they cause any abdominal discomfort?

3. **Personal habits**–Do you drink alcohol? If yes, how often and how many drinks do you have? Do you smoke cigarettes? If yes, how many a day and for how many years have you smoked? Do you eat raw or undercooked foods, such as sushi or eggs? Do you use any illicit drugs currently or in the past? If yes, what are they and how often do you use them? Where have you recently traveled?

    What type of work do you do? Are you exposed to any solvents or chemicals at work?

4. **For older adults**–Do you shop for your own food and prepare it yourself? Do you eat alone or share meals with someone? Have you had recent appetite changes? Do you experience constipation? If yes, how do you treat it?

Objective Information

Equipment Needed

Adequate lighting, exposing only the abdomen; Stethoscope; soft centimeter ruler to measure abdominal girth; skin marking pen; and a small pillow to place under patient's knees to relax the abdominal muscles.

Assessment Techniques

Inspection, auscultation, percussion, and palpation.

The abdominal assessment begins with inspection and proceeds to auscultation so there is no change in bowel sounds. Percussion and palpation of the abdomen increases peristalsis causing an artificial increase in bowel sounds. Percussion is performed after auscultation followed by light and then deep palpation.

Physical Examination

Inspection

The patient is in a supine position with a pillow under the knees bending the knees to relax the abdominal muscles. Have the patient empty the bladder before the examination. Inspect the abdomen for contour, symmetry, skin coloration, lesions, rashes, scars, hair distribution, and abnormal movements, such as pulsations or peristalsis. Mild pulsation in the upper abdomen near the costal angle (over the abdominal aorta) may be seen in slender patients.

Inspect the perianal and sacrococcygeal area for redness of the skin, ulcers, lesions, fissures, swelling, rashes, or dimpling of hair. Ask the patient to tighten the external anal sphincter and note the tone.

Auscultation

Lightly place the diaphragm of the stethoscope on the abdomen at the RLQ and progress to the RUQ, LUQ, and LLQ (see Figure 9-3). Listen for 1-5 minutes for bowel sounds in each quadrant distinguishing pitch, intensity, and frequency of the sounds. Auscultate with the bell of the stethoscope over the aorta (midline upper abdomen), renal (bilaterally in the upper abdomen, near the costal angle), and iliac and femoral (lower quadrants between umbilicus and groin) arteries noting any bruits (swishing sounds).

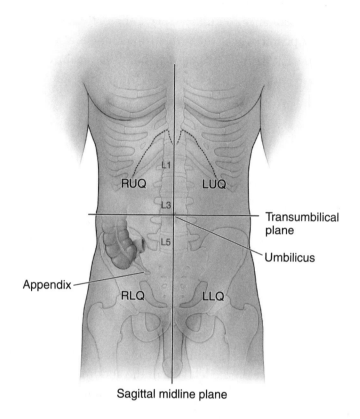

FIGURE 9-3 • Abdominal quadrant partitioning.
(Reproduced with permission from Morton DA, Foreman KB, Albertine KH: *The Big Picture: Gross Anatomy.*
New York, NY: McGraw-Hill; 2011. Figure 7-1A)

Percussion

Percuss the abdomen in the same sequence as auscultation noting change in pitch. If the patient is experiencing abdominal pain, assess that quadrant last. Percuss for the size of the liver at the right midclavicular line tapping over the lungs and proceeding downward toward the liver, listening for a change from lung resonance to dullness over the liver and mark the spot. Then percuss the abdomen moving upward from the waist, listening for tympany over the intestines to dullness over the liver and mark that spot. Measure between the two marks. The normal adult liver is approximately 8-11 cm in men and 6-9 cm in women at the midclavicular line and 6-8 cm in men and 4-6 cm in women at the midsternal line.

Percuss for spleen borders working along the left midaxillary line, starting at the lowest intercostal space above lower costal margin or 10th rib noting changes from lung resonance to dullness. Have the patient sit up and perform indirect percussion posteriorly at the level of the kidneys at the costovertebral angle (CVA) at the 12th rib by placing one hand flat against the back at the level of the 12th rib and strike that hand with the medial side of closed fist on the other hand.

Palpation

Using the same sequence as auscultation, perform light palpation first by depressing about 1 cm, while using a gentle rotation of the fingertips. Next, perform deep palpation by pressing about 5-8 cm deep using the same sequence as above. If the patient is experiencing abdominal pain, assess that quadrant last. Bimanual palpation can be utilized placing one hand on top of the other. Note the size, consistency, tenderness, or mobility of any masses.

Palpate the liver by placing the left hand under the patient's back and pressing under the rib cage on the right side of the abdomen with the right hand pointing the fingertips toward the patient's face. Ask the patient to breathe deeply.

Palpate the spleen by pressing your right hand under the patient's back and pressing under the rib cage on the left side of the abdomen with your left hand pointing the fingertips toward the patient's left shoulder. Ask the patient to breathe deeply.

Palpate the kidneys by placing one hand under the patient's flank and press with the other hand firmly on the abdomen, pressing the two hands together. Repeat on the other side.

Palpate the aorta by placing two fingertips lateral to midline above the umbilicus and press firmly.

Palpate the bladder starting at the suprapubic area moving upward toward the umbilicus.

Expected Findings

Inspection

Inspection of the abdomen reveals the contour to be: flat, scaphoid, rounded, distended, or protuberant.

The skin is evenly pigmented with equal symmetry on both sides of the abdomen. There are no scars, rashes, or lesions. The umbilicus is midline with equal hair distribution and no abnormal movements noted. A flat or rounded abdomen is usually noted. The external anal sphincter is closed tightly.

Auscultation

Normal bowel sounds occur sporadically and are heard as gurgling sounds at a rate of 5-30 per minute. No bruits are heard over the vascular areas.

Percussion

Tympany, a low-pitched, drum-like sound is predominant over the abdomen with dullness heard over the spleen and liver. The normal liver span is 6-12 cm with variations based on body size and gender. Males and those with a long torso may have a wider liver span. Normal spleen width is about 7 cm. Indirect percussion of the CVA angle reveals pressure but no pain.

Palpation

Slight tenderness may be found over the bladder, sigmoid colon, and ovaries. The liver, kidneys, bladder, and spleen are not commonly palpated. The lower edge of the liver should feel smooth and firm. The spleen is normally non-palpable. Palpation of the aorta reveals a regular pulse and is about 2-3 cm in width.

Abnormal Findings

Inspection

A scaphoid abdomen may be seen in a patient with progressive disease or malnutrition and an abdomen may be distended with fluid (ascites), air or gas, obesity, pregnancy, feces, or a tumor.

Asymmetry may be seen with a tumor or mass, organ enlargement, hernia, or bowel obstruction.

Abnormal skin changes include redness that may indicate inflammation; pale, tight skin with abdominal distention of ascites; scars from earlier surgeries; silvery lines called striae indicating prolonged stretching of the skin. Intraabdominal bleeding is indicated by the presence of Cullen sign (ecchymotic discoloration around the umbilicus) or Grey Turner sign (ecchymosis in the flank area).

A protrusion of the umbilicus could indicate an umbilical hernia (abnormal opening in abdominal wall), or may be a normal variant.

Loss of hair on the abdomen or abnormal hair distribution can be associated with an endocrine abnormality.

Pulsations across the abdomen can indicate hypertension, aortic aneurysm, or visible peristalsis.

Auscultation

Abnormal bowel sounds are hypoactive with decreased peristalsis and hyperactive with increased peristalsis. Hyperactive bowel sounds that are loud gurgling sounds are called borborygmi. A bruit over an artery could indicate turbulent blood flow due to narrowing of the vessel lumen.

Percussion

An area of dullness where tympany is expected may indicate a mass, distended bladder, or enlarged liver (hepatomegaly) or spleen (splenomegaly). An abnormal liver span may indicate atrophy of the liver, liver tumor, cirrhosis, or liver abscess. An abnormal spleen span may indicate enlargement of the spleen (splenomegaly) from trauma or infection. Positive pain over the CVA area can indicate kidney inflammation.

Palpation

Abnormal findings include masses; guarding (protection of the area by splinting or moving); rigidity (increased firmness of the abdomen); tenderness, pain, or rebound (increase in pain when quickly releasing pressure on the abdomen). A wider than normal pulsation of the aorta may indicate an aneurysm. A distended bladder is firm and tender to touch and can extend to the umbilicus.

Special Tests for Ascites

Fluid Wave

With the patient lying supine, ask the patient or another healthcare provider to place one hand in the middle of the abdomen and place the other hand on the same side of the abdomen while firmly tapping on the other side (see Figure 9-4A). A positive fluid wave of ascites will be felt on the stationary hand.

Shifting Dullness

With the patient lying supine, percuss from the umbilicus to the patient's side

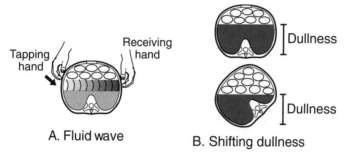

FIGURE 9-4 • Key sign ascites.
(Reproduced with permission from LeBlond RF, DeGowin RL, Brown DD: *DeGowin's Diagnostic Examination*, 9th edition. New York, NY: McGraw-Hill; 2008. Figure 9-21C&D.)

and note the change from tympany to dullness (see Figure 9-4B). Mark the spot. Next, have the patient turn on their side. Percuss again moving up from the bed or examining table, noting the level of dullness. A higher level of dullness reveals a shift of fluid in the abdomen. This shifting level of dullness is positive for fluid in the abdomen of greater than 500 mL.

Special Tests for Appendicitis (Inflamed Appendix)

Rebound Tenderness
Place one hand perpendicular to the abdomen and press firmly on the RLQ and release the hand quickly. Ask the patient, when the most pain was elicited: on pressing or on releasing the hand? A positive finding is pain upon release of the examiner's hand and can indicate peritoneal inflammation.

Referred Rebound Tenderness or Rovsing Sign
Palpate deeply in the LLQ in a similar manner as explained above and quickly release the pressure. Pain upon release of pressure indicates possible peritoneal inflammation and possible appendicitis.

Iliopsoas Sign
With the patient lying supine, have the patient lift the right leg straight up and then let the examiner push against the anterior right thigh while the patient resists lowering the leg. Pain in the RLQ indicates a positive sign and possible inflamed appendix.

Obturator Sign

With the patient lying supine, the examiner rotates the flexed hip and knee internally and then externally. Pain in the RLQ indicates a positive finding and may indicate appendicitis or abscess.

Special Test for Cholecystitis (Inflamed Gallbladder)

Murphy Sign

While palpating deeply in the RUQ toward the liver ask the patient to inhale deeply. The presence of pain and stopping of inspiration is a positive test and may indicate an inflamed gallbladder.

Age-Related Changes

Pediatric

In infants, the liver is more likely to be palpated and the urinary bladder is higher in the abdomen than in the adult. In childhood, the abdominal organs may be palpated easily due to the abdominal muscles being less developed than in adulthood. Specific questions to the mother or caregiver of the infant and child include: Is the infant breastfed or bottle fed? How many times a day do the diapers need to be changed? How many are wet each day and how many bowel movements occur? Does the child eat a variety of foods? For the adolescent, ask about diet and exercise patterns and recent weight loss or gain. Ask the adolescent about self-image and assess for risk of anorexia nervosa or obesity.

Geriatric

It is important to ask the older adult who does the food shopping and who prepares food. Assess risk of nutritional deficiencies based on income or food preferences. Age-related changes to the abdominal system include: decreased salivation and a decreased sense of taste (loss of sensation of bitter, sour and salty, whereas sweet sensation is relatively preserved); increased chance of GERD due to a weaker lower esophageal sphincter; drug metabolism in the liver is slower due to a decreased blood flow in the liver (40% by the age of 80 years); and an increased risk of gallstones in overweight females over the age of 40 years. Peristalsis slows with aging increasing the risk of constipation. Assess all older adults for constipation and ask about bowel movements, water, and fiber intake. Adipose fat moves to the abdomen in postmenopausal females due to the lack of estrogen and older sedentary men tend to gain weight in the abdomen. Muscle tone of the abdominal wall muscles is decreased, enhancing the protuberance of the abdomen as people age.

Cultural Considerations

Several ethnicities have lactose intolerance: East Asians, Africans, Ashkenazi Jews, and people of Mediterranean descent. It is important to ask about reactions to dairy foods. Patients who avoid dairy foods have a risk of calcium deficiency and osteoporosis. Gastric cancer rates are higher among Japanese and Eastern Asians. Ask the patient about use of antacids that might be masking stomach discomfort associated with gastric cancer. Gallbladder cancer rates are highest among American Indians and those of Hispanic descent. Chinese men have high mortality rates from liver cancer. Colorectal cancer is high among all ethnicities and all patients should be encouraged to have a screening colonoscopy at the age of 50 years. Obesity rates are increasing in the USA and other countries. The risk of having diabetes is highest in Asians, Hispanics, and African Americans who are obese. Mexican Americans and African Americans have increased rates of obesity putting them at risk for type II diabetes and other diseases.

CASE STUDY

Mary Jones is a 41-year-old female with complaints of RUQ abdominal pain. Ms Jones is 5 feet 3 inches and weighs 175 lb with a BMI of 31 and is of African descent. The patient states the pain is commonly felt "after eating fried foods." She commonly eats three meals a day: breakfast (cereal with juice and coffee); lunch (a sandwich, cookies, and ice tea); dinner (meat, potatoes or rice, vegetables with butter, white bread, and ice cream at night for dessert). Ms Jones lives with her husband and three children and works part-time as a receptionist.

REVIEW QUESTIONS

1. **The examiner performs Murphy sign on the above patient. The correct technique is:**

   A. place one hand perpendicular to the abdomen and press firmly on the RLQ and release the hand quickly.

B. with the patient lying supine, the examiner rotates the flexed hip and knee internally and then externally.

C. with the patient lying on the left side, percuss from the umbilicus to the patient's side and note the change from tympany to dullness.

D. Palpate by placing the left hand under the patient's back and pressing under the rib cage with the right hand pointing the fingertips toward the patient's face.

2. **Murphy sign is a test to assess for:**

   A. appendicitis.

   B. ascites.

   C. cholecystitis.

   D. kidney infection.

3. **Ms Jones has a BMI of 31 which is classified as which of the following:**

   A. Normal weight.

   B. Overweight.

   C. Obese.

   D. Underweight.

4. **Gastric cancer rates are highest among which of the following ethnicities?**

   A. Japanese.

   B. American Indians.

   C. Africans.

   D. Italians.

5. **The stomach, spleen, and pancreatic body and tail are located in which of the following areas of the abdomen?**

   A. RUQ.

   B. LUQ.

   C. RLQ.

   D. LLQ.

6. **Where would the healthcare provider preparing to palpate the bladder on a patient who has recently urinated, begin palpating?**

   A. Right lower quadrant (RLQ).

   B. Umbilical area.

   C. Suprapubic area.

   D. Epigastric area.

7. **Why should the healthcare provider auscultate the abdomen before palpating or percussing the abdomen?**
   A. Bowel sounds can be increased with palpation.
   B. Palpating the abdomen first could decrease bowel sounds.
   C. Inspection of the abdomen should reveal peristaltic waves.
   D. Fluid in the abdominal cavity can interfere with auscultation.

8. **A patient is complaining of difficulty when swallowing liquids. This is documented as:**
   A. indigestion.
   B. dysphagia.
   C. nausea.
   D. cramping.

9. **The healthcare provider discovers an asymmetrical abdomen in the above patient, Ms Jones. What can this indicate?**
   A. Malnutrition
   B. Hernia
   C. Ascites
   D. Aortic aneurysm

10. **Which of the following is an age-related change to the abdominal system that one might observe in a geriatric patient?**
    A. Change in number of taste buds.
    B. Peristalsis slowing causing constipation.
    C. Adipose tissue decreasing in abdominal area.
    D. Nutritional deficiencies in all elderly patients.

ANSWERS

1. D.
   A. Rebound tenderness
   B. Obturator sign
   C. Shifting dullness

2. C.
   A. Rebound tenderness, referred rebound tenderness, iliopsoas, and obturator sign test for appendicitis.
   B. Fluid wave and shifting dullness test for ascites.
   C. Positive CVA tenderness can indicate kidney inflammation with a kidney infection.

3. C. Obese.
    A. Normal weight is a BMI of 18.5-24.9.
    B. Overweight is a BMI of 25-29.9.
    C. Obese is a BMI of 30 or greater.
    D. Underweight is a BMI of less than 18.5.

4. A. Gastric cancer rates are higher among Japanese and Eastern Asians.

5. B. The stomach, spleen, pancreatic body and tail, as well as the left kidney, left adrenal gland, left ureter, splenic flexure of colon, and transverse descending colon are located in the LUQ.

6. C. The bladder that is not distended is located in the suprapubic area. If the bladder is distended, it can be palpated above the suprapubic area to the umbilicus.

7. A. The abdominal assessment begins with inspection and proceeds to auscultation so the healthcare provider does not change bowel sounds. Percussion and palpation of the abdomen increases peristalsis causing an artificial view of bowel sounds.

8. B. Dysphagia is difficulty swallowing food or liquids. Indigestion is discomfort before or after eating. Nausea is a sensation to vomit, and cramping is a diffuse, dull pain.

9. B.
    A. A scaphoid abdomen can be seen with malnutrition.
    B. A hernia can be seen with an asymmetrical abdomen.
    C. Abdominal distention with pale, tight skin is seen with ascites.
    D. Pulsations across the abdomen can be seen with an aortic aneurysm.

10. B. Peristalsis slows with aging increasing the risk of constipation.

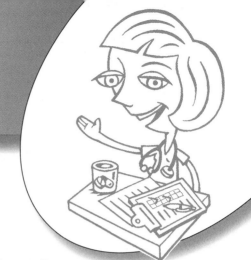

Assessment of the Musculoskeletal System

> ## KEYWORDS
>
> Bursa
> Cartilaginous joint
> Fibrous joint
> Footdrop
> Hyperextension
>
> Osteoblasts
> Periosteum
> Spastic hemiparesis
> Synovial joint
> Temporomandibular joint (TMJ)

Introduction

The musculoskeletal system is composed of the bones, joints, and muscles which serve to support the body and protect the vital organs. On movement, the musculoskeletal system provides stability for the body. The musculoskeletal system also provides support to stand erect and covers the vital body organs, for example: the brain, spinal cord, heart, and lungs. The bones have essential metabolic functions of calcium regulation and the formation of blood cells in the bone marrow.

Review of Anatomy and Physiology

Bones

The skeletal system consists of the bones, cartilage, and ligaments. The ligaments join bones to other bones at the joints. A joint is the place where a bone or cartilage meets another bone. Bones are connected to muscles by tendons. Ligaments and tendons are composed of dense connective tissue that serves to support joints. Bone is a connective tissue of which there are two types: compact bone is hard and compact and forms the outer layer of bone, whereas spongy bone is lighter but has strong tensile strength to support the weight of the body and is found on the inside. Bone tissue is constantly being formed and broken down. The osteoblasts build bone and secrete bone matrix. The osteoclasts reabsorb bone matrix. The osteocytes are mature bone cells. The periosteum is a membrane that covers the bones and provides nourishment via blood vessels.

The skeletal system is composed of: the axial skeleton, consisting of the bones of the skull, thorax, and vertebral column; and appendicular skeleton, consisting of the bones of the upper and lower extremities (see Figure 10-1).

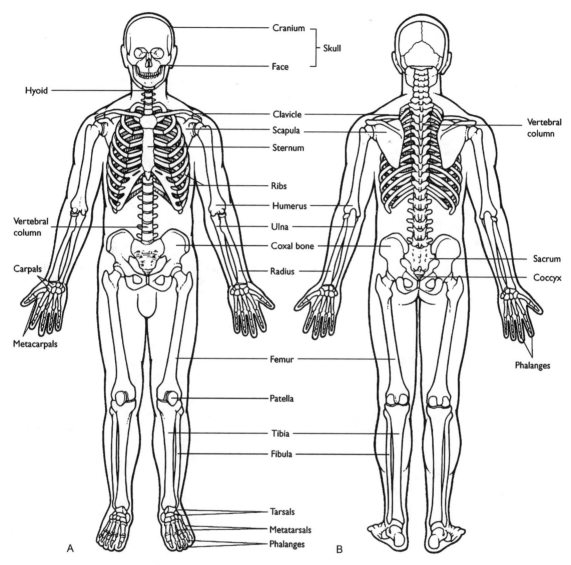

FIGURE 10-1 • Axial and appendicular skeleton.
(Reproduced with permission from Hall SJ: *Basic Biomechanics*, 5th edition. New York, NY: McGraw-Hill; 2007. Figure 4-3.)

Joints

A joint is the place where two bones or cartilage meet and is freely movable, provide slight movement, or are unmovable or fixed. Freely movable joints are called synovial joints where the bone ends are separated by a joint cavity that contains synovial fluid that provides lubrication for the joint (see Figure 10-2). The joint is supported by: the joint capsule that surrounds the joint and consists

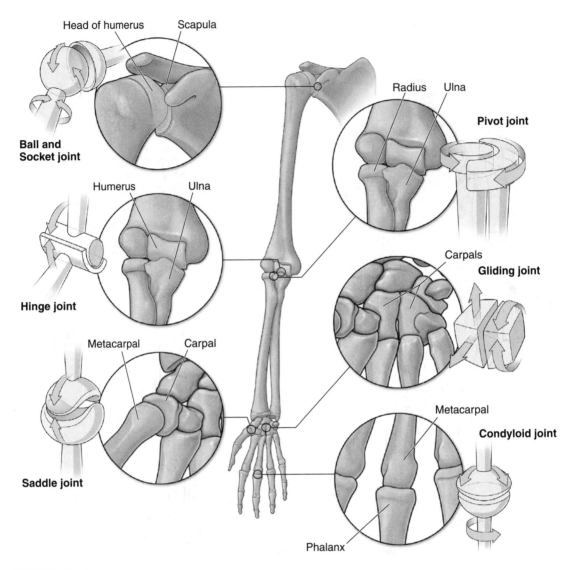

FIGURE 10-2 • Examples of a synovial joint.
(Reproduced with permission from Dutton M: *Dutton's Orthopaedic Examination, Evaluation, and Intervention*, 3rd edition. New York, NY: McGraw-Hill; 2012. Figure 1-3.)

of a fibrous layer; ligaments that extend between the bones; and tendons that attach to muscles. Synovial joints are located at the wrist, elbows, shoulder, knees, and ankles. Joints providing slight movement are called cartilaginous joints, and are located between the sternum and ribs and the symphysis pubis. Joints that are immovable are called fibrous joints, and are joined by dense connective tissue or bone, for example, the sutures in the skull. Some joints contain bursa (a sac containing synovial fluid) or tendon sheaths (tube-like bursa that wrap around tendons) at areas where pressure is exerted. Bursa and tendon sheathes help prevent friction. On injury, bursa can become inflamed causing pain and limited movement of the joint.

Muscles

The skeletal muscles produce body movement, maintain body position, and stabilize joints. The other muscles are cardiac muscle (involuntary muscles that contract the heart) and smooth muscle (involuntary muscles found in the hollow organs of the body).

Skeletal muscles will be discussed because they are the muscles involved in physical assessment (see Figure 10-3 and Table 10-1).

Subjective Information

Interview

The interview of a patient for the musculoskeletal system focuses on activities of daily living (ADLs) and functional assessment, as well as specific questions about the bones, joints, and muscular function. It is important to remember to ask questions about the patient's medical history, present concerns, family history, and lifestyle.

Review of Systems (ROS)

Ask the patient specific questions related to the musculoskeletal system. Are you having any pain in your bones, joints, or muscles? Describe the pain—is it throbbing, sharp, or dull, and does it occur with exercise or at rest? Can you point to the area of pain? Does it occur in a specific bone or joint and does it occur on both sides of the body (bilaterally)? How long does the pain last and what relieves the pain? What treatments have you tried to relieve the pain and do they work? Do you have pain in a specific bone or joint and is it affected by movement? Do you experience stiffness or limited movement of any joints? Have you experienced any trauma to the bones, joints, or muscles? If yes, has this affected the function? Have you noticed any swelling or redness of any joints and do they feel warm or hot at any time? Do you have any deformities of the bones or joints and is this related to trauma? Do you experience

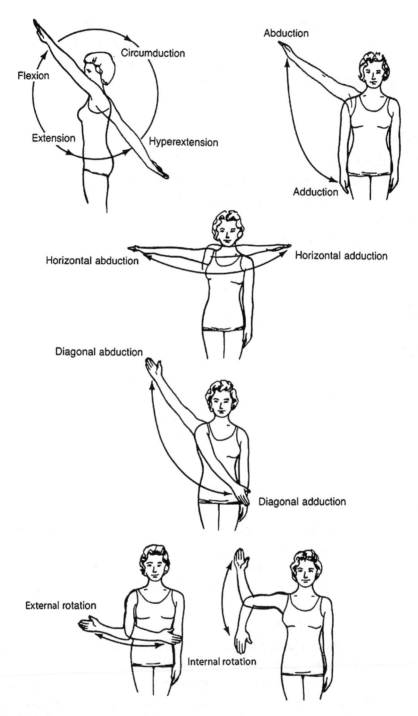

FIGURE 10-3 • Examples of skeletal muscle movements.
(Reproduced with permission from Hamilton N, Weimar W, Luttgens K: Kinesiology: *Scientific Basis of Human Motion*, 11th edition. New York, NY: McGraw-Hill; 2008. Figure 5-10.)

TABLE 10-1 Skeletal Muscle Movements	
Abduction	Movement of an extremity away from the midline of the body.
Adduction	Movement of an extremity toward the midline of the body.
Circumduction	Moving the arm in a circular movement by means of the shoulder joint.
Elevation	Moving a part of the body upward.
Depression	Moving an elevated part of the body downward.
Inversion	Moving the sole of the foot inward and medially.
Eversion	Moving the sole of the foot outward and laterally.
Flexion	Bending an extremity at the joint and bring the bones closer together.
Plantar flexion	Extending the ankle and pointing the toes.
Dorsiflexion	Flexing the ankle and moving the toes toward the ankle.
Extension	Straightening the extremity at a joint.
Hyperextension	Extension beyond 180 degrees
Pronation	Moving the forearm, so that the palm of the hand is downward.
Supination	Moving the forearm, so that the palm of the hand is upward.
Protraction	Moving a body part forward and parallel to the ground.
Retraction	Moving a body part backward and parallel to the ground.
Rotation	Turning of a bone along its own axis.
Internal rotation	Toward the midline.
External rotation	Away from the midline.
Opposition	Touching the thumb to the tip of the other fingers.

numbness or tingling in your extremities? If yes, where does it start—the fingers or toes, and where does it stop?

Associated Symptoms

1. **Fever**–Do you have a fever or elevated temperature? Do you feel excessively warm at any time of the day?
2. **Rash**–Do you have any rashes, hives (itchy red rash), or a butterfly-type rash across your nose and cheeks?
3. **Fatigue**–Have you felt fatigue or weakness? Have you had a persistent stiffness in your neck?

Risk Factors Related to the System

The risk factors for patients with an increased risk of developing musculoskeletal disease are: family history of arthritis, repetitive movements that are work or sports related, obesity, gender, and age.

Risk Evaluation

1. **Family history**–Does anyone in your family have a history of any bone, joint, or muscle deformities? Does anyone in your family have a history of osteoarthritis, rheumatoid arthritis, scoliosis, or osteoporosis? If yes, at what age did it develop, how was it diagnosed, and how is it being treated? What treatments have been successful?

2. **Personal history**–Have you experienced any trauma to the bones, joints, or muscles? For example, a fracture, dislocation, or muscle sprain or strain. If yes, at what age did it occur? How was it treated? Did you have surgery to correct any injuries? Was any hardware placed in your body to stabilize the injury? Do you have any residual deformities or limited movement related to the injury? Do you experience pain at the injury site? If yes, does the pain occur with movement or at rest? Does swelling redness or heat occur at the site of the injury? How do you treat the pain?

Do you have a history of any bone, joint, or muscle diseases? For example: scoliosis or spinal deformities, osteoarthritis, rheumatoid arthritis, osteomyelitis, osteopenia, or osteoporosis? If yes, describe any pain experienced with the condition. When it occurs, how severe the pain is, where is the pain located, how long does it last, and what are the treatments that are successful? Has this condition interfered in your lifestyle? What changes have you made to adjust to the condition? Has the condition added stress to your life and how do you cope with the added stress of a musculoskeletal disorder?

Have you ever fallen? Do you use a device to assist walking, for example, a cane or walker?

Do you have a history of any systemic disease that causes bone or joint pain? For example, systemic lupus erythematosus, Lyme disease, or psoriatic arthritis.

3. **Personal habits**–Do you engage in any personal habits to support your bones, joints, and muscles? Do you perform weight-bearing exercises? Describe your exercise routine: How long does the routine last and how

many days a week do you exercise? Do you participate in any sports? If yes, how often and do you wear any protective gear? What is your occupation? Does your job require any heavy lifting? What type of shoes do you wear? Do you wear special footwear (orthotics) devices in your shoes?

Have you recently gained more than 10 lb? Describe your diet. Do you eat any foods with calcium? For example, dairy products, lentils, or beans? Do you take calcium or Vitamin D supplements? How much and how often? How much time do you spend in the sun daily?

For postmenopausal women–Have you had a bone density scan? What were the results? Do you take calcium and Vitamin D supplements? Do you perform weight-bearing exercises? Describe the routine.

Do you take any medications? Certain medications can cause arthralgia (joint pain) or myalgia (muscle pain). Do you smoke cigarettes or drink alcohol? Smoking tobacco and heavy alcohol use may place the patient at risk for osteoporosis. The patient who drinks 2-3 ounces of alcohol daily does not absorb calcium from the intestines adequately and the liver cannot activate Vitamin D, which is important for calcium absorption.

For older adults–It is important to assess the patient's ADLs. Do you need assistance with any of the following activities: bathing, toileting, brushing your teeth or hair, shaving, getting dressed, walking, or climbing stairs? Do you use any assistive devices? It is also important to ask about independent ADLs (IADLs). Do you need assistance with preparing food, shopping for food, or eating food? Who cares for your home? For example, cleaning, doing laundry. Do you need assistance with using the telephone, talking, or writing?

Objective Information

Equipment Needed

Flexible tape measure–To measure circumference of extremities and/or length of the arms or legs.

Goniometer–An instrument that measures the angle where the joint can flex or extend.

Assessment Techniques

Inspection and palpation.

Physical Examination

Inspection

In a head-to-toe fashion, inspect each muscle group and joint starting at the midline of the body and proceeding to the outside evaluating the extremities last (proximal to distal). Inspect muscles and overlying tissue of each joint for changes in color of the skin, redness, ecchymosis, swelling, or obvious joint or bone deformities. Compare each side of the body noting symmetry of the muscles and joints.

Palpation

In a head-to-toe fashion, palpate each muscle group and joint starting at the midline of the body and proceeding to the outside evaluating the extremities last (proximal to distal). Palpate for joint or bone deformities, nodules, temperature and moisture of the skin, and swelling or masses. Ask the patient if palpation reveals pain or tenderness.

Range of Motion (ROM)

Ask the patient to move each muscle group and joint as the healthcare provider inspects and palpates. Support the joint at rest and do not forcibly move the joint if the patient is not able to fully move the joint. Repeat all movements against resistance.

Head and Neck

Temporomandibular Joint (TMJ) (see Figure 10-4)

Inspect: Inspect in front of the tragus and ear.

Palpate: The healthcare provider places the third and fourth fingers anterior to the tragus as the patient opens the mouth to the widest possible position, moves the joint side to side, and protrudes and retracts the jaw. The mouth should open 3-6 cm wide and 1-2 cm from side to side, and is able to protrude and retract without resistance.

Abnormal findings: Crepitus, pain or tenderness, or decreased range of motion (ROM) of the TMJ joint, which could indicate dysfunction of the TMJ joint.

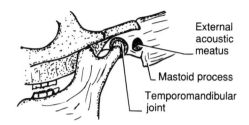

FIGURE 10-4 • Anatomy of the TMJ.
(Reproduced with permission from LeBlond RF, DeGowin RL, Brown DD: *DeGowin's Diagnostic Examination,* 9th edition. New York, NY: McGraw-Hill; 2008. Figure 7-28.)

Spine

Inspection of the spine with the patient in a standing position and the health-care provider standing behind the patient.

Cervical (see Figure 10-5)

Inspect: Inspect the cervical spine for a concave curvature and obvious deformities. The head is erect.

Palpate: Palpate all spinous processes of the cervical spine for pain or tenderness and the vertebra prominens (C7) at the base of the neck. Normal findings include firm muscles, with no pain or tenderness.

ROM: Ask the patient to flex the head forward and then bend the head back. Normal flexion is 45 degrees and normal extension is 55 degrees. Ask the patient to touch each ear to the shoulder to test lateral bending. Normal lateral bending is 40 degrees. Ask the patient to turn the head to the right and left to test rotation. Normal rotation is 70 degrees. Repeat all movements against resistance.

Thoracic and Lumbar (see Figure 10-6)

Inspect: Inspect the thoracic spine for a convex curvature and the lumbar spine for a concave curvature and obvious deformities. Inspect for symmetry of the shoulders, scapula, and hips.

Palpate: Palpate all spinous processes of the thoracic spine for pain or tenderness.

ROM: Ask the patient to bend forward and attempt to touch the toes. Normal forward flexion is 75-90 degrees. Ask the patient to extend the

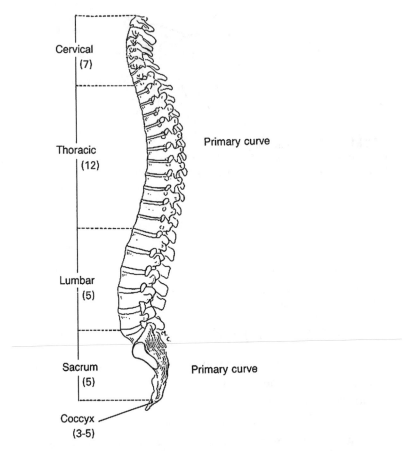

FIGURE 10-5 • Lateral view of the spinal column.
(Reproduced with permission from Hamilton N, Weimar W, Luttgens K: *Kinesiology: Scientific Basis of Human Motion*, 11th edition. New York, NY: McGraw-Hill; 2008. Figure 9-1.)

spine back. Normal extension is 30 degrees. Next, ask the patient to bend to the right and left side and twist from side to side. Normal lateral flexion is 35 degrees and normal rotation is 30 degrees. Repeat all movements with resistance. All spinous processes should feel firm, smooth, and free of pain or tenderness. Normal finding is no decrease in ROM with resistance.

Abnormal findings: Abnormal findings of the spine include pain, tenderness or muscle spasm, and decreased ROM, which could indicate muscle strain or fracture of a spinous process. Spinal pain that radiates to the extremities associated with reduced ROM could indicate degenerative disc disease or spinal cord compression. Associated symptoms of fever, chills, and headache could indicate meningitis.

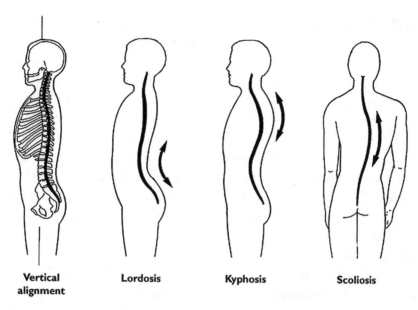

| Vertical alignment | Lordosis | Kyphosis | Scoliosis |

FIGURE 10-6 • Abnormal spine curvatures.
(Reproduced with permission from Hall SJ: *Basic Biomechanics*, 5th edition. New York, NY: McGraw-Hill; 2007. Figure 9-12.)

ALERT

Abnormal structural changes include:

Kyphosis: An exaggerated thoracic curvature that could indicate osteoporosis.

Scoliosis: Lateral curvature of the spine with an exaggerated convexity of the thoracic and/or lumbar spine.

Lumbar lordosis: An exaggerated lumbar curvature often seen in pregnancy or abdominal obesity.

Arms

Shoulders and Elbows

Inspect: Inspect bilateral shoulders and elbows for symmetry, color of the skin, lesions, masses, or obvious deformities.

Palpate: Palpate for masses, swelling, or increase in temperature of the skin. Ask the patient if pain or tenderness is experienced while palpating. Palpate the muscles of the arm and shoulder, as well as the acromioclavicular and glenohumeral joints.

ROM: Ask the patient to bring the arms forward, bending at the elbows, and then extending the arms behind the body. Normal flexion of the arms is 180 degrees and hyperextension is 50 degrees. Next, have the patient reach both arms overhead with elbows extended and both palms touching overhead. Normal abduction is 180 degrees. Ask the patient to bring both arms with elbows extended back to the midline of the body. Normal adduction is 50 degrees. Ask the patient to bring both hands behind the head with the elbows flexed and then behind to the lower back. Normal external and internal rotation is 90 degrees. Ask the patient to flex and extend the elbow. Normal flexion of the elbow is 160 degrees with 0 degree of extension.

Abnormal findings: Unsymmetrical or flattened shoulders, swelling, masses or pain, and tenderness with palpation or movement. Decreased ROM, muscle weakness, or muscle atrophy can be seen with rotator cuff tear, and increased temperature of the skin, redness, and swelling can be seen with bursitis of the olecranon process. Tenderness upon palpation of the elbow can be seen with epicondylitis from repetitive movement.

Wrist, Hands, and Fingers

Inspect: Inspect the wrist, hands, and fingers for symmetry, size, shape, color of the skin, and swelling.

Palpate: Palpate the wrist and each joint of the fingers for pain or tenderness, nodules, and crepitus of the joints.

ROM: Ask the patient to bend the wrist downward and back upward. Normal flexion and hyperextension are 90 degrees. Next ask the patient to hold the wrist straight and bend laterally and medially. Normal radial (medial) deviation is 20 degrees and normal ulnar (lateral) deviation is 55 degrees. Ask the patient to bend the fingers downward and upward. Normal flexion of the fingers is 90 degrees and hyperextension is 30 degrees. Ask the patient to spread the fingers apart, bend the fingers into a fist, and touch the thumb to the fifth finger. The fingers should be able to abduct 20 degrees and return together (adduction) and normal thumb flexion is 50 degrees.

Abnormal findings: Pain with ROM, tenderness upon palpation, or decreased ROM can indicate arthritis or muscle or joint disease.

> ### ALERT
>
> **Test for carpal tunnel syndrome:**
> **Phalen Test:** Ask the patient to flex the wrist and place the dorsum of both hands together, and hold this position for 1 minute. An abnormal finding is pain, numbness or tingling of the wrist.

Tinel sign: Tap on the inner aspect of the wrist over the median nerve. An abnormal finding is pain, numbness, or tingling of the wrist.

Bouchard nodes and Heberden nodes are hard, painless nodes seen with patients who have osteoarthritis of the hands. Bouchard's nodes are in the proximal joints and Heberden's nodes develop in the distal joints.

Hips and Knees

Inspect: While the patient is in a standing position, inspect the iliac crests and buttocks for symmetry, and both knees for shape, size, symmetry, and swelling.

Palpate: Palpate for crepitus, pain or tenderness, warmth, and mobility.

ROM: Ask the patient to lie supine and raise the right leg while it is extended. Normal hip flexion with the knee straight is 90 degrees. Next bend the knee to the chest. Normal hip flexion with the knee bent is 120 degrees. Next ask the patient to straighten the leg and bring it away from the body (abduction) and then to the midline of the body (adduction). Normal abduction of the leg is 45 degrees and normal adduction is 30 degrees. Next rotate the knee and leg internally and externally. Normal external rotation is 45 degrees and normal internal rotation is 40 degrees. Ask the patient to bend the knee toward the buttocks and then straighten the knee. Normal knee flexion is 120-130 degrees and normal extension is 0 degree. Ask the patient to hyper-extend the leg, with the patient being prone or in standing position. Normal hyperextension of the leg is 15 degrees.

Abnormal findings: Pain or tenderness on movement or palpation or decreased ROM may indicate muscle or joint disease of the hips or knees.

ALERT

Bulge Test: Massage the medial aspect of the knee toward the upper thigh and then press on the lateral side of the knee, while looking for a bulge on the medial side. A bulge on the medial side of the knee is found with a small amount of fluid in the knee joint.

Ballottement Test: Hold the knee firmly with your thumb and index finger and press the knee toward the femur with your other hand. Movement of the patella or a click is a sign of a large amount of fluid in the knee joint.

> **McMurray Test:** Place your hand on the patient's flexed knee and rotate the leg laterally and extend the knee slowly. Repeat rotating the leg medially and extending the knee slowly. Clicking of the knee or pain may indicate a torn meniscus.

Ankles and Feet

Inspect: Inspect the ankles and feet while the patient is sitting, standing, and ambulating, for alignment, shape, symmetry, and swelling.

Palpate: Palpate the ankles, feet, and toes for pain or tenderness, edema, nodules, crepitus, warmth, or increase of temperature of the skin.

ROM: Ask the patient to dorsiflex the foot by turning it upward and then plantar flex the foot by turning it downward. Normal dorsiflexion of foot and ankle is 20 degrees and normal plantar flexion of the foot and ankle is 45 degrees. Next, ask the patient to perform inversion of the foot by turning the soles inward and eversion of the foot by turning the soles outward. Normal inversion is 30 degrees and normal eversion is 20 degrees. Next, ask the patient to turn the foot outward for abduction and inward for adduction. Normal abduction is 10 degrees and normal adduction is 20 degrees. Next, have the patient flex the toes under the foot and extend them upward. Normal flexion and extension of the toes is 40 degrees.

Abnormal findings: Pain or tenderness upon movement or palpation or decreased ROM may indicate muscle or joint disease of the ankles, feet, or toes.

Common abnormalities of the foot include: feet with high arches or no arches (flat feet), thickened skin at pressure points (calluses), warts, and plantar warts (occur under the skin). A painful, tender, inflamed great toe could indicate gouty arthritis. Pain or tenderness is seen with osteoarthritis and nodules and pain are seen with rheumatoid arthritis. A deviated great toe and overlapping of the second toe is seen with an inflamed bursa (bunion).

Ambulation and Gait

Inspect: Ask the patient to stand and walk across the room while the health-care provider observes the position of the feet, the posture, arm swing, and stability of ambulation. The patient should be able to stand on both toes and both heels. The toes should point forward and arms should swing in a fluid fashion in the opposite direction of the legs. The posture should be erect and the weight evenly distributed.

Abnormal findings: The patient cannot stand on either their heels or toes and weight is not evenly distributed. Shoes are worn unevenly revealing an uneven gait.

ALERT

Common gait abnormalities

Footdrop: Foot slaps downward with each step seen with disease of lower motor neurons.

Spastic hemiparesis: The patient drapes the toe or leg of one side of the body and holds a flexed arm of the same side close to the body, seen with patients with a cerebral vascular accident.

Cerebellar ataxia: A wide, staggering, unsteady gait seen with alcoholic intoxication and cerebellar disorders.

Parkinsonian gait: A shuffling stiff-looking gait with the patient hunched over, seen in patients with Parkinson disease.

Scissors gait: The patient overlaps the thighs with each step and has short, stiff steps, seen with partial paralysis of the legs.

Expected Findings

Inspection

Inspection reveals even pigmentation over all the joints with no color changes, redness, ecchymosis, or pallor. No swelling or masses are evident. The joints and bones do not have any obvious deformities.

Palpation

Palpation reveals smooth skin with even pigmentation, no obvious deformities, masses, or nodules. Skin is warm and dry without swelling, and on palpation the patient does not complain of pain or tenderness.

Range of Motion

Reveals full expected ROM of the joint without pain, tenderness, or crepitus.

Abnormal Findings

Inspection

Redness and swelling can indicate effusion (an increase of fluid in the joint), or thickening and inflammation of the lining (synovium) of the joint cavity.

Ecchymosis, purplish discoloration can indicate bleeding into the subcutaneous tissue of the joint.

Joint deformities can indicate subluxation (misalignment of the joint), dislocation (complete separation of the two bones that form a joint), ankylosis (decreased or complete immobility of a joint due to fusion of the bones of the joint, commonly caused by trauma, disease, or chronic inflammation), joint contracture (loss of passive ROM of a joint due to structural changes from disease, trauma, muscle wasting, or immobilization of the joint).

Palpation

Skin over muscles or joints that is hot to the touch and reveals swelling indicates inflammation.

Painful muscles and joints to touch could indicate inflammation.

Crepitus, a grating sound and/or feeling of a joint on movement could indicate loss or damage of cartilage.

Range of Motion

Limited ROM of a joint less than the expected range.

Pain or tenderness with ROM of a joint.

Age-Related Changes

Pediatric

The cartilaginous skeleton forms *in utero* by 3 months and continues to develop after birth forming new bones. Bone is deposited around the shaft of bones during childhood. Bones lengthen at the growth plates (epiphyses) by depositing cartilage at the end of the long bones. The epiphyses are commonly closed by 21 years of age. Muscle fibers are all present at birth and continue to lengthen during childhood. During adolescence, muscular growth is increased due to the secretion of growth hormones. Scoliosis (a lateral curvature of the spine) commonly becomes evident in adolescence, due to the rapid growth of the spine. Muscle strength and size is determined by genetics, nutrition, and exercise.

Geriatric

The elderly patient is at risk for osteoporosis, which is a condition where the bone density is lost over time. Osteoblasts decrease production with age, thereby decreasing the number of osteocytes; however, osteoclasts continue to reuptake bones. This results in bone with decreased density and strength. Kyphosis, an exaggerated curvature of the thoracic spine, can develop in the older patient with osteoporosis.

ALERT

The risk factors for osteoporosis are:

Age: As one ages, the risk of developing osteoporosis increases.
Gender: Females have thinner and lighter bones.
Ethnicity: Caucasians and Asians have a higher incidence of hip fractures from osteoporosis.
Body weight: Petite women have less bone to lose.
Family history: Family and personal history of fractures increases the risk.
Postmenopause: Decreased estrogen enhances the ability of osteoclasts to absorb bone.
Diet: A diet lacking sufficient calcium and Vitamin D (calcium helps build bone and Vitamin D helps with the absorption of calcium).
Personal habits: Smoking decreases bone density and alcohol decreases the absorption of calcium and Vitamin D.
Medications: Corticosteroids decrease the levels of estrogen in women, decrease the amount of calcium absorbed, and increase the calcium excretion through the kidneys.

The elderly patient will often complain of losing height. As one ages, water is lost from the intervertebral disks which causes loss of height. Joints become less flexible and cartilage loses water content. Tendons and ligaments lose flexibility and become stiff, decreasing ROM of the joints. Muscle loss occurs especially after the age of 60 years and it is prudent for the healthcare provider to educate the elderly patient to have an adequate intake of calcium, Vitamin D, and to perform weight-bearing exercises. Exercise and proper nutrition helps to delay the process of osteoporosis and increases skeletal mass. Bony prominences become more obvious as one ages as subcutaneous fat is distributed in the abdomen and hips and away from the periphery and face. The loss of subcutaneous fat over bony prominences such as the hips and pelvis puts the bedbound elderly patient at risk of bedsores (decubitus ulcers). The contour of muscles becomes more distinct and tendons more visible.

Cultural Considerations

There are several differences that can be found in the musculoskeletal system. Africans can have a larger gluteal prominence than Caucasians providing an appearance of increased lumbar lordosis. Children of African descent have a higher bone density than children of Caucasians. Adolescents of African descent have a 10-15% greater bone density than Caucasians. African and Hispanics have a decreased risk of fractures than Caucasians. Women of all races have been found to have a peak of spinal bone mass by the age of 33 years that gradually decreases with age. Bone density is higher in men than women. Hispanics have a slightly higher bone density as compared with Caucasians. Therefore, Caucasian women have a higher incidence of fractures of the spine and hip.

CASE STUDY

Ms Cho is an 80-year-old patient, who came to the clinic today complaining of low back pain as well as pain in her knees and hips upon awakening. The patient lives alone on the second level and must walk up the stairs to her apartment. Ms Cho prepares all of her own meals but stated that food "does not taste as good as it used to." She admits to the healthcare provider that she often does not eat yogurt or milk-based products, because they upset her stomach. The patient is of Asian descent and is 5 feet tall and weighs 110 lb. Her BMI is 21.5. The healthcare provider notes that the patient has kyphosis.

REVIEW QUESTIONS

1. The healthcare provider understands that one of the risk factors for osteoporosis is which of the following:

   A. small stature.
   B. BMI greater than 20.
   C. diet high in calcium.
   D. exercising three times a week.

2. The healthcare provider is assessing the patient's risk factors for osteoporosis. What additional information should the healthcare provider obtain in the above case study?

   A. Does your apartment house have an elevator?
   B. Have you gained weight recently?
   C. Do you take a multivitamin?
   D. Have you had many fractures of bones?

3. Which of the following absorbs bone?

   A. Osteoblasts
   B. Osteocytes
   C. Osteoclasts
   D. Periosteum

4. The healthcare provider asks the patient to perform flexion of the knee to assess range of motion (ROM). The normal ROM of flexion of the knee is:

   A. 90 degrees.
   B. 120 degrees.
   C. 150 degrees.
   D. 40 degrees.

5. The healthcare provider is preparing to assess abduction of the legs. What should the healthcare provider instruct the patient to perform?

   A. Ask the patient to lie supine and raise the right leg while it is extended.
   B. Ask the patient to straighten the leg and bring it away from the body.
   C. Ask the patient to bend the knee to the chest.
   D. Ask the patient to straighten the leg and bring it to the midline of the body.

6. Ms Cho is complaining of joint pain. The healthcare provider would document this finding as:

   A. arthralgia.
   B. myalgia.
   C. cephalgia.
   D. neuralgia.

7. Why is it important for the healthcare provider to assess the amount of alcohol intake for a patient at risk for osteoporosis?

   A. Alcohol interferes with the production of osteoblasts.
   B. Alcohol increases the excretion of calcium via the kidneys.
   C. Alcohol decreases the absorption of calcium and Vitamin D.
   D. Alcohol intake can change the number of osteoclasts.

8. The healthcare provider is examining Ms Jones' fingers and assesses redness, swelling, and coolness to the touch over the fourth right finger. What could this indicate?

   A. Bleeding into the subcutaneous tissues.
   B. Fusion of the bones of the joint.
   C. Inflammation of the joint.
   D. An increase of fluid in the joint.

9. The healthcare provider assesses Ms Jones and documents kyphosis of the spine. What is the definition of kyphosis?

   A. Lateral curvature of the spine.
   B. An exaggerated lumbar curvature.
   C. An exaggerated thoracic curvature.
   D. Reduced ROM of the spine.

10. The healthcare provider is assessing the patient's independent activities of daily living (IADLs). Which of the following should the healthcare provider ask the patient?

   A. "Are you able to do your own laundry?"
   B. "Do you take any medications?"
   C. "Do you need assistance in dressing?"
   D. "Do you have a history of fractures?"

ANSWERS

1. A. Ms Cho is at risk for osteoporosis because of her short stature, ethnicity, age, gender, and body weight. A BMI of 20 is normal and not a risk factor for osteoporosis, and a diet high in calcium and exercise are recommendations to prevent osteoporosis and are not risk factors.

2. D. A personal history of fractures or a family history of fractures increases the risk of a patient having osteoporosis. An elevator would be helpful if the patient complains of joint pain, but if the patient can walk the stairs daily mild exercise might help prevent osteoporosis. A recent weight gain would not increase the risk of osteoporosis. However, a 24-hour nutritional recall would provide information regarding the patient's nutritional status and calcium intake. A multivitamin does not provide sufficient amounts of calcium and Vitamin D to prevent osteoporosis.

3. C. Bone tissue is constantly being formed and broken down. The osteoblasts build bone and secrete bone matrix. The osteoclasts reabsorb bone matrix. The osteocytes are mature bone cells. The periosteum is a membrane that covers the bones and provides nourishment via blood vessels.

4. B. The normal knee flexion is 120-130 degrees.

5. B. Abduction moves an extremity away from the median of the body. A is testing hip flexion, C is testing hip flexion, and D is testing adduction.

6. A. Myalgia is muscle pain, cephalgia is a headache, neuralgia is pain that follows the path of a nerve.

7. C. The healthcare provider should assess the amount of alcohol intake by asking about the number of alcoholic drinks the patient has in a day and the amount in each glass, because alcohol intake can decrease the absorption of calcium and Vitamin D.

8. D. Redness and swelling of a joint can indicate effusion (an increase of fluid in the joint). Purplish discoloration can indicate bleeding into the subcutaneous tissue of the joint. Skin over muscles or joints that is hot to the touch and reveals swelling indicates inflammation. Decreased or complete immobility of a joint may be due to fusion of the bones of the joint.

9. C. Kyphosis is an exaggerated thoracic curvature. Scoliosis is a lateral curvature of the spine with an exaggerated convexity of the thoracic and/or lumbar spine. Lumbar lordosis is an exaggerated lumbar curvature. A reduced range of motion (ROM) of the spine could indicate degenerative disease.

10. A. Independent activities of living (IADLs) include: shopping, preparing, and eating food, and caring for the home. Activities of daily living (ADLs) include: bathing, toileting, brushing teeth or hair, shaving, getting dressed, walking, or climbing stairs. Asking about medication use and a history of fractures would assess osteoporosis risk.

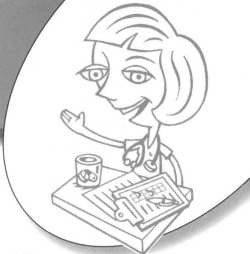

chapter 11

Assessment of the Nervous System

LEARNING OBJECTIVES

After reviewing this chapter, the learner will be able to:

1. Identify important anatomic landmarks of the neurologic system.
2. Discuss the appropriate information to gather during an interview.
3. Demonstrate a physical assessment of the neurologic system.
4. List normal physical assessment findings.
5. Describe abnormal physical assessment findings.
6. Discuss the age-related differences related to the neurologic system.

KEYWORDS

Anosmia	Meninges
Deep tendon reflex	Parietal lobe
Dermatomes	Romberg test
Dysmetria	Somatic system
Graphesthesia	Stereognosis
Hypothalamus	

Introduction

The nervous system is a highly complex, extremely vital component for the functioning of the human body. Essentially, almost all of our bodily functions, both voluntary and involuntary, are controlled through the proper functioning of the nervous system. It is composed of both the central and peripheral nervous systems. The central nervous system includes the brain and spinal cord. The peripheral nervous system includes the nerves throughout the body that transmit signals to and from the central nervous system. A complete assessment will include detailed observation of motor, sensory, behavioral, and cognitive functions. Additionally, a comprehensive interview will provide the healthcare provider with the proper tools to better understand the potential factors that may be associated with abnormalities.

Review of Anatomy and Physiology

Central Nervous System

The brain and the spinal cord make up the central nervous system and are responsible for maintaining the overall coordination of the body. The skull and vertebrae create a protective vault. The central nervous system is protected by the cerebrospinal fluid and a network of membranes known as meninges, which consist of the dura mater, arachnoid mater, and pia mater (see Figure 11-1).

The brain consists of three main divisions: the cerebrum, the cerebellum, and the brainstem. The brain is essentially supplied with a symmetric blood supply that consists of the internal carotid arteries, the vertebral arteries, and the basilar arteries. This bilateral blood flows through the circle of Willis as it distributes its oxygen-rich blood to the different areas of the brain.

The cerebrum is divided into two hemispheres with multiple, identical lobes on each side. The outer layer, or cortex, controls higher level functioning, such

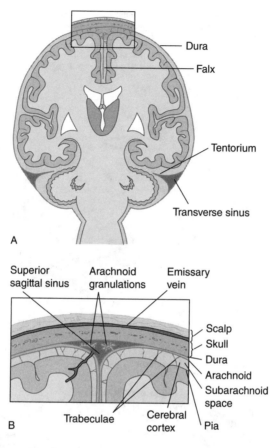

FIGURE 11-1 • Illustration of meninges.
(Reproduced with permission from Waxman SG: *Clinical Neuroanatomy*, 26th edition. New York, NY: McGraw-Hill; 2010. Figure 11-5.)

as reasoning, thought, memory, sensation, and a variety of voluntary movements. These lobes include the frontal lobe, the parietal lobe, the occipital lobe, and the temporal lobe (see Figure 11-2). The frontal lobe is associated with many personal behavior controls, emotions, and impulse control. The parietal lobe is primarily responsible for sensory control, proprioception, as well as some of the visual, olfactory, and auditory sensations. The occipital lobe is situated in the posterior aspect of the brain and is typically identified by the occipital groove in the posterior area of the skull. It is primarily responsible for interpreting visual data. The temporal lobe functions mainly in the processing and interpretation of auditory stimuli.

The cerebellum is located just inferiorly to the occipital lobe of the cerebrum. It functions mainly to assist in the coordination of voluntary muscle movement, though it is entirely subconscious. It also promotes balance and posture.

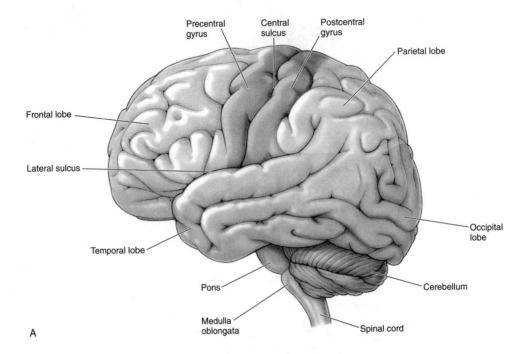

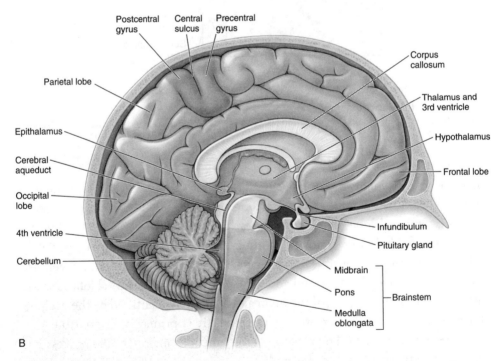

FIGURE 11-2 • Divisions of the brain.
(Reproduced with permission from Morton DA, Foreman KB, Albertine KH: *The Big Picture: Gross Anatomy.* New York, NY: McGraw-Hill; 2011. Figure 16-1.)

The brainstem is the innermost brain core that consists of the medulla oblongata, the pons, and the midbrain. The medulla has a crucial role in many autonomic functions, such as respiration and heart function. The midbrain terminates in the thalamus and hypothalamus, which maintains consciousness, alertness, and temperature and pain perception. Finally, the 12 cranial nerves, which are peripheral nerves, have fibers that originate in the brainstem.

The spinal cord is the highway that allows for the transmission of motor and sensory impulses to and from the brain. It is protected by the vertebral column, which is divided into the cervical (neck), thoracic (chest), lumbar (mid back), and sacral (pelvic) areas. It originates at the medulla oblongata and terminates at the cauda equina ("horse's tail") at the level of the second lumbar vertebrae (L2). It is composed of horn-shaped gray matter containing nerve cell bodies. Additionally, it contains myelin-coated white matter that allows for propagation of impulses along the ascending and descending tracts. The ascending tracts include the dorsal and spinothalamic tracts and mediate sensory signals that are responsible for pinpoint discrimination, proprioception (sense of spatial orientation), deep pressure, temperature, and pain. The descending tracts are responsible for transmitting impulses from the brain to the periphery to promote or inhibit motion and maintain posture.

Peripheral Nervous System

The peripheral nervous system is a complex network of nerves that serve as a transportation network for transmitting impulses to and from the central nervous system via the afferent and efferent nerve fibers. The spinal and cranial nerves constitute the peripheral nervous system and can be divided into the somatic and autonomic systems. The somatic system functions as voluntary control and innervates the skeletal muscles in the body. The autonomic system regulates unconscious activities in the body and plays an integral role in maintaining overall balance, or homeostasis, in the body. This system innervates the smooth, or involuntary, muscles of the body.

Spinal nerves are peripheral nerves that originate along the length of the spinal cord. There are 31 pairs of nerves that are named for the area of the spine from which they originate. These include cervical, thoracic, lumbar, sacral, and coccygeal, and contain both motor and sensory fibers. The sensory and motor functions of particular areas of the skin are regulated by single segments of certain spinal nerves. These areas are referred to as dermatomes and are able to transmit signals from adjacent dermatomes (see Figure 11-3).

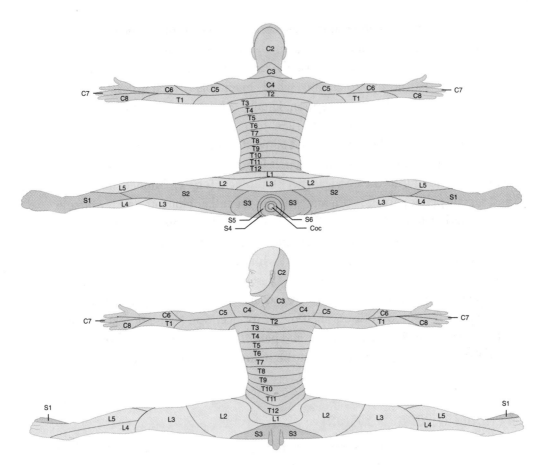

FIGURE 11-3 • Sensory dermatomes.
(Reproduced with permission from Tintinalli JE, Stapczynski JS, MA OJ et al: *Tintinalli's Emergency Medicine: A Comprehensive Study Guide*, 7th edition. New York, NY: McGraw-Hill; 2011. Figure 158.1-1.)

Cranial Nerves

There are 12 cranial nerves that originate from the brain rather than the spinal cord (see Figure 11-4). These nerves can have either motor or sensory functions; some have both motor and sensory functions. See Table 11-1 for the description of these nerves, as well as their function and location.

Subjective Information

When assessing the nervous system, the practitioner will need to conduct a clear and thorough interview of the patient. Often, a detailed interview may uncover crucial pieces of information that will help to determine subtle changes in the nervous system. Changes in mental status may also signal neurologic pathology.

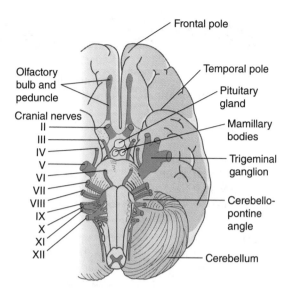

FIGURE 11-4 • Illustration of the cranial nerves.
(Reproduced with permission from Waxman SG: *Clinical Neuroanatomy*, 26th edition. New York, NY: McGraw-Hill; 2010. Figure 8-1.)

Interview

The interview of the patient can lead to discovery of vital information that will often guide clinical decision making and treatment plans. It is important to remember that the patient with neurologic deficits may have difficulty with memory (recollection) and communication. Therefore, the interviewer must ask straightforward, clear questions with all patients. It is often helpful to restate the patient's answer to ensure accuracy. Additionally, the interviewer must take the time to elaborate on any deficiencies or complaints to discriminate between simple, chronic ailments and potentially serious issues. In order to do this, care should be taken to always identify aggravating and alleviating factors, methods used to manage symptoms, onset of symptoms, and level of debilitation from symptoms. A comprehensive history should also be established.

Review of System (ROS)

The ROS for the neurologic system should focus on symptoms that might be related to issues of the neurologic system. However, as the neurologic system affects every other system in the body, the questions may be more general in nature when compared to performing an ROS for other organ systems. The patient should be questioned about headaches, including severity, frequency, timing, and effective measures to treat their headache. It should be established

TABLE 11-1 Cranial Nerves

Cranial Nerve	Function	Test	Expected Findings	Abnormal Findings
I Olfactory	S (sensory)	Odor discrimination	Correct identification of different odors	Anosmia—decreased or loss of smell bilaterally with allergies, tobacco, or drug use
II Optic	S	Visual acuity Visual fields Optic disc	Equal and consensual pupils Symmetric eye movements	Visual field loss with lesions
III Oculomotor	M (motor)	Extraocular movements (EOMs) Pupil constriction Eye opening	Eye movement toward upper, outer, lower outer, and upper inner areas	Unequal pupil constriction or eye opening Ptosis
IV Trochlear	M	EOM (downward, inward)	Eye movement toward the tip of the nose	Unequal eye movement
V Trigeminal	B (both sensory and motor)	Facial sensation (ophthalmic, maxillary, mandibular) Corneal reflex Masseter strength Lateral movement of jaw	Symmetric tone. Symmetric discrimination for sensations	Muscle atrophy Jaw deviation Fasciculations Impaired sensations Lack of corneal reflex
VI Abducens	M	EOM Lateral deviation	Lateral eye movement	Unequal movement
VII Facial	B	Facial symmetry (expression, mouth, closing eye) Strength Taste (anterior two–thirds tongue = sweet and salty) Labial speech sounds (m, b, p)	Facial symmetry Clear speech annunciation	Tics Unusual or asymmetric facial movements Difficulty annunciating labial sounds

(Continued)

TABLE 11-1 Cranial Nerves (*Continued*)				
Cranial Nerve	**Function**	**Test**	**Expected Findings**	**Abnormal Findings**
VIII Vestibulocochlear	S	Hearing—whisper test Bone and air conduction of sound—Rinne test Balance (Romberg test)	Correct identification of whispered words Air conduction	Altered ability to detect sounds
IX Glossopharyngeal	B	Swallow and gag reflex Palate elevation (Ahh!) Voice quality/ hoarseness Sensation— posterior tympanic membrane and auditory canal Taste discrimina- tion (posterior tongue = sour and bitter)	Gag reflex Equal elevation of soft palate Proper taste identification of posterior tongue	Loss of gag reflex Unequal palate elevation Poor identification of taste on posterior tongue
X Vagus	B	Assess symmetry in palate and uvula Assess swallowing Assess guttural speech	Symmetry of movement of soft palate	Asymmetric tonsilar or soft palate movement Deviation of uvula (Hoarse or brassy voice with vocal cord issues; nasal twang with weak soft palate)
XI Spinal accessory	M	Test trapezius strength through shoulder shrug Test sternomastoid muscle through lateral head movement	Bilaterally equal muscle strength	Muscle weakness or atrophy
XII Hypoglossal	M	Inspect tongue position and movement Evaluate lingual speech sounds (l, t, d, n)	Central protrusion of tongue	Lateral tongue deviation

if there is severe neck stiffness also, as this may indicate inflammation of the meninges or meningitis. Red flags for headache symptoms would be systemic symptoms (fever, pregnancy, and cancer), new onset of headaches, onset over the age of 50 years, change in headache pattern, neurologic symptoms or headaches that follow trauma or worsen with the Valsalva maneuver.

The patient should be questioned about visual, hearing, and taste changes, and if there have been any recent changes in swallowing or speech.

It is important to determine any history of head trauma, as well as potential loss of consciousness, vision, or headaches that correlate with trauma. Seizure history, including auras, frequency, and type of seizure must be determined.

Sleep patterns, behavioral changes, changes in alertness, and focus should also be established. It is important to determine if there are any balance disturbances, neuralgias, numbness or tingling to specific areas of the body, or loss of motor control or tone in any part of the body. It is crucial to gain as much detailed information about any of these findings to determine if the cause is neurologic in nature, or can be attributed to some other disease or culprit. Cerebellar function should be established through careful questioning related to balance and coordination. The patient should be asked about leaning toward one side when ambulating and about any recent falls. Dysmetria refers to the inability to control range of motion. Episodes of dizziness, lightheadedness, and syncope need to be established, and causes include neurologic, cardiac, and inner ear disturbances. When asking about episodes of dizziness, the healthcare provider needs to establish whether the person felt as if they were spinning, or if the room seemed to be spinning. The latter is a sign of vertigo and may be associated with inner ear infections, labrynthitis, or neurologic dysfunction.

Risk Factors Related to the System

There are many risk factors that may cause neurologic impairment. These factors range from environmental factors to drug usage to medical history. It is important to establish history of earlier strokes, transient ischemic attacks (TIAs), meningitis, spinal cord injury, and cardiac/circulatory disorders.

Drugs alter the individual's mental and neurologic status. Care should be exercised to determine the type, amount, and frequency of both drug and alcohol use. Consideration should also be given to the patient's family history, including alcoholism, muscular dystrophy, Huntington chorea, seizure disorders, migraines, mental retardation, dysfunction of the thyroid, diabetes, hyper- or hypotension, and Tay-Sachs disease.

Exposure to potential environmental hazards, such as lead, insecticides, chemicals, extensive exposure to heights or water, and arsenic should be established. It is essential to determine the individual's work history, even if remote, to determine potential exposure to any of the above hazards. Finally, consideration must be given to other preexisting medical problems, or risk factors, that may increase the chance of a stroke. These risk factors include hypertension, dyslipidemia, obesity, sedentary lifestyle, tobacco use, increased stress, atrial fibrillation, oral contraceptives, sickle cell anemia, diabetes, and congenital anomalies.

Objective Information

Equipment Needed

- Penlight
- Tongue blade
- Sterile needle or paper clips
- Tuning forks
- Familiar objects, to be used for discrimination
- Cotton wisp
- Reflex hammer
- Common odors (such as vanilla, peppermint, coffee) for cranial nerve testing
- Samples of warm and cold water, if testing temperature discrimination

Assessment Techniques

Inspection
Palpation
Percussion
Auscultation

Mental status examination—It is imperative to establish a baseline cognitive assessment on patients. A mini mental status examination, such as the Folstein Mini Mental Status Examination, can be easily administered to patients to screen for cognitive dysfunction. Areas of orientation, registration, recall, attention, calculation, language, repetition, and complex commands are tested.

Physical Examination

An organized, sequential assessment must be performed due to the complexity of the neurologic system. A cephalo caudal approach is typically used. The cranial nerves are typically the first to be examined and should be examined as discussed in the above table.

Cerebellar Function

Careful assessment of the patient's fine motor skills and coordination are important components of the neurologic assessment. Motor function can be assessed by having the patient rapidly alternate movements by rapidly patting each knee with their hands, alternating the palmar and dorsal aspects. Movements should remain smooth and rhythmic and should not be jerky, discoordinated, or clonic. Also, they should be able to efficiently alternate between touching their nose and the interviewer's finger with their index finger. This, too, should be smooth and accurate.

Balance can be assessed through a variety of examinations. The Romberg test should be performed on the patient by asking them to stand with their arms at their side and eyes open. They should then close their eyes and the interviewer will assess for stability of stance. It is acceptable to have mild swaying, but staggering, losing balance, or falling is considered abnormal findings. Testing for pronator drift is accomplished by having the patient stand with arms outstretched and then closing their eyes. The arms should remain parallel to the floor, despite the loss of visual cue. The healthcare provider should remain close to the patient for both the Romberg and the pronator drift test, in case balance is lost. The patient should also be examined for balance by asking them to hop on one foot with their eyes open for 5 seconds then repeat on the other foot for 5 seconds. They should be able to do this without having to touch the elevated foot to the ground. Finally, the patient should be asked to walk around without shoes, alternating their eyes open and closed. They should be able to ambulate smoothly, without gait disturbances, regardless of whether their eyes are open or closed. They should also be able to tandem walk, or walk heel to toe, in a forward and backward straight line, while continually maintaining heel-to-toe contact. Lateral staggering, use of arms for balance, or falling are unexpected findings and could indicate cerebellar dysfunction.

Sensory Function

Testing for temperature, pain, and vibratory discrimination will assess sensory function. When completing a comprehensive assessment, it is important to test each sense bilaterally at each major peripheral nerve ending, typically in the extremities. The healthcare provider should test these senses with the patient's eyes closed and with progressive stimulation. Careful note should be taken for the amount of stimulation needed for the patient to identify and discriminate the characteristic and location of these tests. It is expected that the patient is able to identify the stimulation at comparable intensities bilaterally, correctly identify the type of sensation experienced (ie, sharp versus dull, hot versus cold), and have appropriate proprioception, or isolate the sensation to the correct body side, location, and proximity related to an earlier sensation. Vibratory discrimination is tested with the use of a low-pitched tuning fork (128 Hz works well). The tuning fork is struck against the provider's hand to cause vibration. The handle of the tuning fork is placed on a bony area (such as a joint) to see if the patient can feel the vibration. This is also checked for symmetry. Occasional placement of the tuning fork should be with a nonvibrating tuning fork to see if the patient can distinguish. Abnormal findings, or findings that differ from the above, should be carefully documented with extent of altered sensation, type of stimulation that was misidentified, and where the sensation is correctly identified again.

Cortical sensation refers to the body's ability to cognitively discriminate and interpret different sensations. Tests to assess for this include two-point discrimination, stereognosis, or the recognition of familiar objects, point location, and graphesthesia, or the ability to identify letters or numbers. Two-point discrimination tests whether the patient can distinguish whether one or two point are making contact. The use of an opened paperclip easily provides both one and two points. The two points need to be at least 5 mm apart in order for most individuals to discriminate. Stereognosis is the ability to identify common objects by touch. Place a coin, key, or paperclip into the patient's hand to see if they can correctly identify the object. Point location is tested by randomly touching different areas on the patient and having the patient identify the area being touched. Graphesthesia is tested by tracing a letter or number on the palm of the patient's hand. The patient should be able to correctly identify what was traced. The tests are completed with the patient's eyes closed.

Reflexes

Deep tendon reflexes are a motor response to a sensory stimulation. A peripheral tendon is stimulated sending a signal to the spinal cord, which causes a reflex response in muscular activity. There is no conscious processing of the stimulus involved in the response. These reflexes can aid in the assessment of the central nervous system of the comatose patient or help to determine the level of spinal cord injury. Intact reflex responses signal normal neuromuscular function in the area being tested. Abnormal findings in deep tendon reflexes can signal neuro-muscular damage. The patient should be relaxed with the limbs supported to accurately assess reflexes. If the patient is holding their limb in a particular position, the inherent muscle tension will prevent the reflex. If you are having difficulty in testing the reflexes, try distraction. Have the patient count out loud or focus on a motor activity in a different area (have them tap their foot while you test a bicep reflex). Reflexes are documented as a number, representing a range from absent (0) to clonus (5+), with 2+ representing normal. (Table 11-3)

Abdominal reflexes are cutaneous reflexes. They are tested by gently stroking the abdomen on an angle from the corner of an outer quadrant toward the umbilicus. Presence of the reflex is normal and will elicit contraction of the underlying muscles, resulting in the umbilicus moving slightly toward the

TABLE 11-2 Testing reflexes		
Reflex	**Assessment**	**Spinal Column Level**
Biceps	Place your thumb over the bicep tendon in the antecubital area and strike your thumbnail with the reflex hammer. Produces elbow flexion (contraction of the biceps brachii muscle)	C5–C6
Triceps	The patient's elbow should be flexed. Tap the tricep tendon, proximal to the elbow on the posterior surface of the arm, with the reflex hammer. Produces elbow extension (contraction of the triceps muscle)	C7–C8
Brachioradialis (supinator)	Tap the lateral forearm about 3 inches (8–10 cm) above the wrist in an adult. Produces mild wrist extension or radial deviation (contraction of the brachioradialis muscle)	C5–C6
Patellar	Tap the patellar tendon (between patella and tibia) while the knee is flexed. Produces forward movement of the lower leg or a slight kick. (contraction of the quadriceps muscle)	L2–L4
Achilles tendon	Gently dorsiflex the foot and tap on the Achilles tendon with the reflex hammer. Produces plantar flexion (contraction of the gastrocnemius muscle)	S1

TABLE 11-3 Grading of Reflexes		
Grade	Response	Finding
0	Absent	Always abnormal
1+	Diminished	May be normal or abnormal
2+	Normal	Normal
3+	Increased	May be normal or abnormal
4+	Hyperreflexive or repeating (clonus)	Always abnormal
5+	Sustained clonus	Always abnormal

direction of the stimulus. Absence of the reflex may be due to a lesion or damage to the motor neurons. The upper abdominal reflexes are innervated by T9-T11 nerve roots and the lower abdominal reflexes are innervated by T11-T12 nerve roots. The reflex may be absent in patients with a history of abdominal surgery, obesity, pregnancy, scoliosis, and in elderly patients.

Age-Related Changes

Pediatric

Assessment of neurologic function is routinely checked at birth, at 3, 6, 12, 18, and 30 months. Behavior, posture, tone, head circumference, cranial nerves, reflexes, and developmental milestones are assessed.

Behavior–Look at the physical activity of the baby.

Posture–Look at the position of the baby, and how they hold their arms and legs.

Tone–Look at the baby's overall muscle tone. Are there active movements of all extremities, only some flexion of the extremities, or is the baby flaccid?

Check arm recoil–How far a baby's arm will bounce back to a flexed position after being extended by the examiner. Assess a square window—how far the baby's hand can be flexed toward the wrist. Check the popliteal angle—how far the baby's knees are extended.

Head circumference–Normal newborn head circumference should be 12.5-14.5 inches (32-37 cm) or slightly larger than the chest circumference. Anterior and posterior fontanels should be noted. The anterior fontanel is diamond shaped and should close by 12-18 months of age. The posterior fontanel is triangular and should close by 2-3 months of age.

Cranial nerves–Cranial nerves can be assessed at the same time as the newborn reflexes.

Cranial nerve II is checked by the baby's response to bright light.

Cranial nerves III, IV, and VI are assessed by eye movement. Checking for doll's eye will assess these cranial nerves—turning the baby's head results in the eyes maintaining the same position of gaze.

Cranial nerves V, VII, IX, X, and XII are involved in eating (sucking and swallowing). Cranial nerves IX and X are also checked by assessing the baby's strength and quality of cry.

Cranial nerve VII is checked by looking at the baby's facial symmetry.

Cranial nerve VIII is checked by the baby's response to sound.

Reflexes–During the first day of life, an assessment is made to evaluate neurologic development and function. Newborn reflexes (or primitive reflexes; see Table 11-4) are typically inhibited or changed within the first year, allowing for a postural reflex system (more mature or secondary reflex) as the central nervous system continues to develop. Presence of primitive reflexes for extended periods may indicate neurologic disorders. Deep tendon reflexes are checked as in adults, but a gentler stimulus is used. Tapping the patellar tendon with the examiner's finger should elicit a response—there is no need to use a reflex hammer on a baby.

Developmental milestones are assessed throughout infancy and childhood to assess for normal development and progression of function.

Geriatric

Some common abnormal neurologic findings found in older adults include a diminished arm swing when walking; decrease in vibration sensation; hyperreflexia in the upper extremities; absence of pupillary response and unequal nasolabial folds.

Cerebrovascular accidents (CVA) are the leading cause of disability and death in older adults. Rapid identification of new-onset neurologic abnormalities can assist in the identification of neurologic injury and result in early access to appropriate care. Neurodegenerative disorders (such as amyotrophic lateral sclerosis) are more common as people age. Radiculopathy is also more common as people age. This is typically due to compression of a spinal nerve root. Older patients are more likely to have osteophyte (bone spur) formation (typically due to arthritis) of bones, which will compress nerve roots. Peripheral neuropathy is more common in older patients and may affect as many as one in five older patients. Diabetes mellitus is a common cause of peripheral neuropathy.

TABLE 11-4 Newborn reflexes			
Reflex	**Duration**	**Stimulus**	**Response**
Moro (startle)	Disappears at 3–4 mo	Loud noise or sudden movement	Startling, arms flail out, then flex toward the body
Blink	Permanent	Puff air into the face or flash of light	Eyes close
Palmar grasp	Lessens at 3 mo, disappears at 1 y	Touch the palm	Hand closes
Rooting	Disappears at 3–4 mo	Stroke the cheek or side of the mouth	Turns toward the stimulus, opens mouth to suck
Sucking	Disappears at 3–4 mo	Touch the lips	Opens mouth and sucks
Asymmetric tonic neck	Disappears by 6 mo	Turn the head to the side (looking toward the shoulder)	Arm and leg will extend on the side the infant is facing and flex on the opposite side
Symmetric tonic neck	Disappears by 6 mo	Flexion or extension of the head	Flexion of head causes flexion of arms and extension of legs; extension of head causes extension of the arms and flexion of the legs
Stepping	Disappears at 3–4 mo	Hold the infant upright with feet touching flat surface	Moves legs quickly, raising one then the other, as if to walk.
Crawl	Disappears at 3–4 mo	Place the infant prone (on stomach) on a flat surface	Moves arms and legs as if to crawl
Gallant	Disappears at 1–3 mo	Holding the infant supported face down, gently stroke along one side of vertebral column from top to bottom	Curvature of trunk toward the stimulated side

Cultural Considerations

There are no significant differences in the incidence or presentation of neurologic disorders. Patients and their families may differ in their tolerance of the physical manifestations of neurologic disorders.

CASE STUDY

Adeline is brought in for evaluation by her daughter. Her daughter is concerned that Adeline experienced an episode where she had a temporary loss of balance, slurred speech, and difficulty moving her right arm. The episode lasted for about 10 minutes and occurred several hours ago. Her daughter wanted to bring her to the hospital at that time, but Adeline refused. The patient states that she feels well now and does not know what all the fuss is about.

REVIEW QUESTIONS

1. **The nervous system is composed of:**
   A. the brain.
   B. the spinal cord.
   C. the peripheral nervous system.
   D. all of the above.

2. **Higher level functioning, such as reasoning, thought, memory, and sensation are controlled in the:**
   A. cerebral cortex.
   B. cerebellum.
   C. brainstem.
   D. hypothalamus.

3. **The ascending tracts within the spinal cord are responsible for:**
   A. mediating the sensory signals responsible for proprioception.
   B. transmitting the impulses to promote motion.
   C. transmitting the signals responsible for maintaining posture.
   D. mediating the impulses that inhibit motion and maintain muscle tone.

4. **Proprioception is best defined as:**
   A. the ability to discriminate two different points of contact.
   B. transmission of impulses from the brain to the periphery to inhibit motion.
   C. the ability to determine one's own position in space and the position of varied body parts relative to other body parts.
   D. the point of spinal cord termination at the level of the second lumbar vertebrae.

5. **Equality of pupillary constriction is controlled by cranial nerve:**
   A. I.
   B. III.
   C. VIII.
   D. XII.

6. Part of the evaluation for Adeline includes performing a Romberg test and checking for pronator drift. An abnormal result in either test would indicate the need for further evaluation of:

   A. mental status.
   B. brainstem activity.
   C. peripheral neuropathy.
   D. cerebellar function.

7. Checking for presence of a patellar deep tendon reflex in Adeline is normal and equal bilaterally. This reflex assesses neuromuscular function at the level of:

   A. C5-C6.
   B. C7-C8.
   C. L2- L4.
   D. S1.

8. Abdominal reflexes are assessed by:

   A. placing your thumb on the tendon in the antecubital area and striking your thumbnail with the reflex hammer.
   B. gently stroking the skin at an angle from the lateral corner toward the center.
   C. deeply palpating the abdomen and quickly releasing the pressure.
   D. deeply palpating in an upward direction just below the right costal margin, while the patient takes a deep breath.

9. A common cause of peripheral neuropathy is:

   A. hyperlipidemia.
   B. diabetes mellitus.
   C. transient ischemic attack (TIA).
   D. osteoarthritis.

10. Adeline is able to correctly identify a paperclip placed in her hand when her eyes are closed. This test is called:

   A. stereognosis.
   B. two-point discrimination.
   C. graphesthesia.
   D. point location.

ANSWERS

1. D. The brain, spinal cord, and the peripheral nervous system are all components of the nervous system.

2. A. The cerebellum controls voluntary muscle movement. The brainstem controls respiration and heart function. The thalamus and hypothalamus control consciousness, temperature, and pain perception.

3. A. The ascending tracts mediate signals that are responsible for pinpoint discrimination, proprioception, pressure, and pain. The descending tracts transmit impulses that promote or inhibit motion and help maintain posture.

4. C. Proprioception is the ability to determine one's own position in space and the position of varied body parts relative to other body parts, a sense of spatial orientation.

5. B. Cranial nerve III controls pupillary constriction, eye opening, and upper and outer and lower and outer eye movements.

6. D. Romberg and pronator drift both assess cerebellar function.

7. C. Bicep and brachioradialis reflexes assess C5-C6. Patellar reflexes assess L2-L4. Achilles reflex assesses S1.

8. B. Gently stroking the abdominal skin from the outer corner of a quadrant toward the center should elicit an abdominal reflex. A strike to your thumbnail while holding your thumb over the tendon in the antecubital space should elicit a bicep reflex. Deep palpation of the abdomen followed by a quick release is the technique used to check for rebound tenderness that can signal peritoneal irritation. Deep, upward palpation below the right costal margin is the technique to assess for Murphy sign, which indicates gallbladder irritation.

9. B. Diabetes mellitus is a common cause of peripheral neuropathy.

10. A. Stereognosis is the ability of the patient to identify common objects by touch. Two-point discrimination is tested by the ability of the patient to differentiate between one and two points of contact. Graphesthesia is the ability of the patient to identify a letter or number traced on their palm. Point location describes the ability of the patient to locate the area being touched.

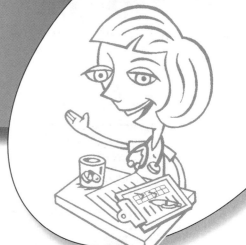

Assessment of the Male Genitourinary System

LEARNING OBJECTIVES

After reviewing this chapter, the learner will be able to:

1. Identify important anatomic landmarks of the male genitourinary system.
2. Discuss the appropriate information to gather during an interview.
3. Demonstrate a physical assessment of the male genitourinary system.
4. List normal physical assessment findings.
5. Describe abnormal physical assessment findings.
6. Discuss the age-related differences related to the male genitourinary system.

KEYWORDS

Benign prostatic hypertrophy (BPH)
Corpus cavernosa
Dysuria
Epididymis
Epispadias

Hypospadias
Inguinal nodes
Lymphatic fluid
Urethra
Varicoceles

Introduction

Disorders involving the male genitourinary tract can affect health status and/or quality of life. Either of these may be very distressing to the patient. Patients and caregivers may feel uncomfortable about discussing issues involving the male genitourinary tract. It is important to make the patient feel at ease in discussing all health-related topics. Healthcare providers may need to overcome their own discomfort in discussing what may be sensitive topics.

Review of Anatomy and Physiology

Kidneys are located high in the posterior part of the abdomen (see Figure 12-1). They are protected from trauma by the lower ribs. The kidneys collect waste materials and excess fluid to produce urine. The urine drains from the kidneys through the ureters. The ureters empty into the bladder. Urine empties from the bladder through the urethra. The urethra in the male patient is approximately 22-cm (8.66-inches) long and is located within the corpus spongiosum. The opening (meatus) of the urethra is found at the tip of the penis. The urethra also allows for the passage of semen during ejaculation. The penis is composed of highly vascular erectile tissue found within two columns, the corpus cavernosa (see Figure 12-2).

The scrotum is a loose pouch of skin which contains two testes, each in its own compartment. The left testis is normally lower than the right testis. They have a rubbery consistency and range in size from 3.5 to 5.5 cm. Testosterone is produced by the testes. Developmental changes in male genitalia during puberty are due to the effects of testosterone. Secondary sexual characteristics are also the result of testosterone. These include development of facial and body hair, deepening of the voice (due to enlargement of the larynx), and muscle development. The testes are also responsible for the production of spermatozoa.

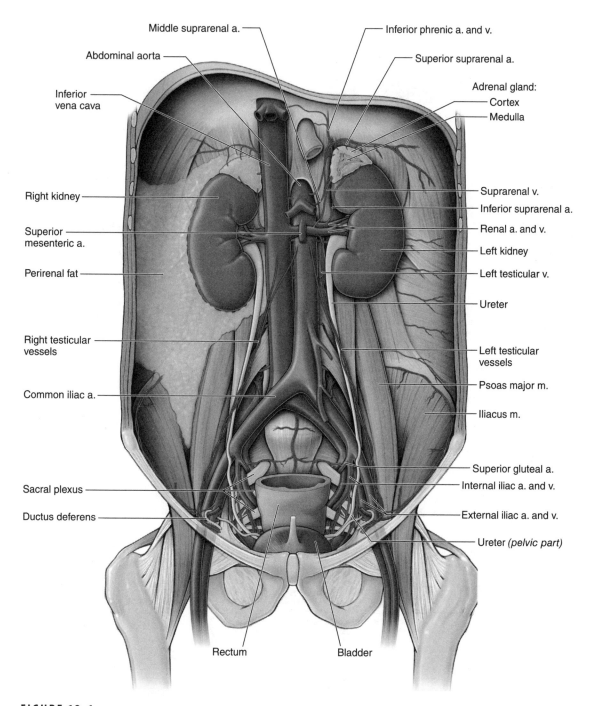

FIGURE 12-1 • Male genitourinary anatomy.
(Reproduced with permission from Morton DA, Foreman KB, Albertine KH: *The Big Picture: Gross Anatomy.* New York, NY: McGraw-Hill; 2011. Figure 11-5.)

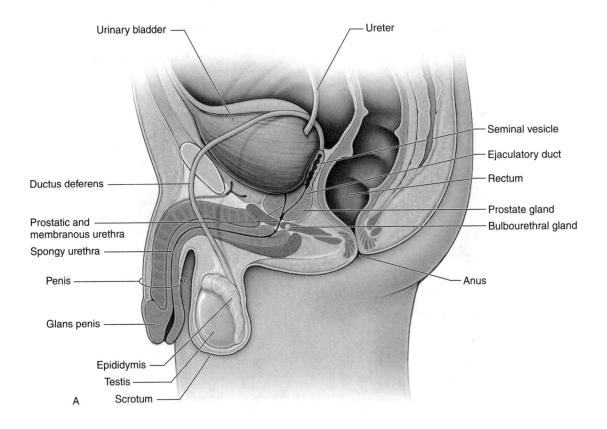

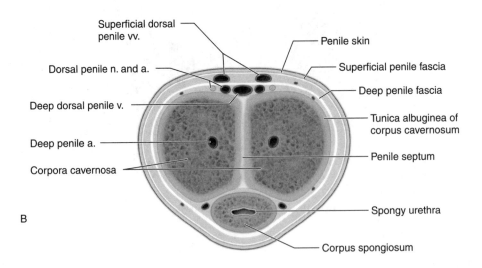

FIGURE 12-2 • Male reproductive system.
(Reproduced with permission from Morton DA, Foreman KB, Albertine KH: *The Big Picture: Gross Anatomy.* New York, NY: McGraw-Hill; 2011. Figure 13-1.)

Attached to the posterolateral area of each testis is the epididymis. Within the epididymis are spermatic ducts where the spermatozoa that have been produced can be stored and allowed to mature fully. The sperm will be transported from the epididymis to the vas deferens, which begins at the epididymis and travels up through the inguinal canal to the abdomen where it meets the seminal vesicle and empties into the urethra. Semen comprises fluids from the vas deferens, the seminal vesicles, and the prostate.

The prostate gland is located beneath the bladder, anterior to the rectum, and encircles the urethra. There is a median sulcus (depression) on the posterior aspect of the gland, which may be palpated through the anterior rectal wall.

Normal male sexual function requires an adequate arterial blood supply, testosterone, and intact nerve functioning, both locally and within the spinal cord. Local vasodilation is responsible for the erection that occurs in response to stimuli.

Lymph nodes drain lymphatic fluid. The inguinal nodes drain from the scrotal skin and penis. These superficial nodes are divided into the vertical and horizontal chains. The vertical chain can be palpated on the medial aspect of the upper thigh near the groin. You can palpate the femoral artery and move 1-2 cm medially to palpate the vertical chain which lies distal to the inguinal crease. The horizontal chain can be palpated at the inguinal crease near the inguinal ligament. The testes drain lymphatic fluid into the abdominal nodes, which are not palpable.

Subjective Information

Interview

Symptoms involving the male genitourinary system may be both concerning and embarrassing for your patient to discuss. Showing compassion for the patient's feelings can help to ease the emotional discomfort the patient may be experiencing.

Review of Systems (ROS)

Ask the patient about any discomfort (dysuria) with urination. If present, ask the patient to describe the sensation: burning, dull ache, sharp pain, etc. Also, determine the timing of the discomfort. Does it occur at the onset of urination, at the end of urination, or does it persist throughout? Discomfort may be associated with infection. Urinary tract infections are more common in women than in men due to the difference in the length of the urethra. The female urethra is approximately 4-cm long and the male urethra is approximately 22-cm long.

Ask about frequency or urgency. More frequent urination and the sudden sensation of the need to urinate can both be signs of infection or irritation of the lower urinary tract structures. Ask the patient about the presence of any flank pain. Pain in the area of the kidneys may be due to infection or kidney stones. Infection of the genitourinary tract is more common in the lower structures (bladder and urethra) than in the kidneys.

Ask about pain in the flank area. Infection may cause discomfort in the posterior upper abdomen, near the junction of the 12th rib and the vertebral column. There may be associated fever, chills, or dysuria with infection. Kidney stones may also cause pain in the flank area. The pain of kidney stones tends to be moderate to severe and occurs intermittently. This pain may radiate to the lower anterior abdomen, groin, scrotal area (in males), or vulvar area (in females).

Inquire about any discharge. Discharge is often associated with infection. The patient may be aware of the discharge, or may have noted staining on the undergarments. Ask about the color, amount of discharge, and any associated symptoms, such as discomfort, fevers, skin lesions, etc. Ask about any prior sexually transmitted infections.

Ask the patient about any discomfort or swelling of the scrotum. Inquire when the patient first noticed the symptoms and if he has noted any alleviation of symptoms with changes in position.

Ask about sexual function. Has the patient noted any change in desire, function, erectile strength, or stamina? Is the patient experiencing any discomfort with ejaculation? Ask if the patient is currently in a sexual relationship. Identify the patient's sexual preference, whether he has sexual relations with women, men, or both. Ask if they engage in vaginal, rectal, and/or oral sexual activity. Ask if the patient engages in safe sex practices. Find out if the patient has any concerns about their sexual health.

Risk Factors Related to the System

Some patients may engage in high-risk sexual behavior. Risk of contracting sexually transmitted infections increases greatly when there is a direct skin to mucous membrane (oral, vaginal, or rectal) contact.

Kidney stones may be due to metabolic problems, which cause a buildup of substances (such as calcium, oxalate, uric acid, or struvite) that can crystallize forming stones. Inadequate fluid intake (less than 1 L/day) contributes to stone formation in patients with a predisposition to kidney stones. Patients with a predisposition to kidney stone formation may develop stones after starting certain medications (thiazide diuretics, topiramate).

Risk Evaluation

Ask the patient about high-risk sexual behavior. Is the patient aware of safe sexual practices, such as the use of barriers (latex condoms or dental dams)? Do they always use a barrier when engaging in oral, vaginal, or anal sex? Is there a history of multiple sexual partners? An increase in the number of partners increases the risk of contracting a sexually transmitted infection. Has the patient begun a new sexual relationship recently? Is there any history of sexually transmitted infections?

Does the patient have a history of urinary tract infections? How often do they occur? Does the patient feel that all symptoms associated with the infection resolve when the infection is treated? Does the patient see a healthcare provider to get treatment when symptoms return? Is the treatment effective?

Patients with a family history of kidney stones are more likely to develop stones themselves. Metabolic disorders (such as gout) and certain medications (such as thiazide diuretics) increase the chances of developing kidney stones.

As men age, they may experience benign prostatic hypertrophy (BPH). Since the prostate gland is located surrounding the urethra at the bladder neck, urinary symptoms develop when the gland is enlarged. The prostate gland enlargement causes lower urinary tract symptoms such as nocturia (getting up at nighttime to urinate), urinary frequency (more frequent need to urinate), urgency (the sensation of having to urinate right away), hesitancy (difficulty initiating urination), dribbling (at the end or after urination), and the sensation of still having a full bladder after urinating.

The risk of prostate cancer increases as men age. The majority of prostate cancers occur in men over the age of 65 years. Family history of prostate cancer increases the likelihood of developing prostate cancer by over 50%. Prostate cancer is more common in North America, northwestern European countries, Australia, and the Caribbean. African American men have a higher risk for developing prostate cancer and are more likely to be diagnosed when the disease is more advanced. Increased intake of a high-fat diet and red meat seems to increase the risk.

Objective Information

Collection of objective information during the physical examination can assist in proper diagnosis of the cause of symptoms.

Equipment Needed

Gloves, penlight.

Assessment Techniques

Inspection, palpation, percussion.

Physical Examination

Inspect the skin of the penis and scrotum for any lesions, areas of excoriation, nits, or lice. If the patient is not circumcised, gently retract the foreskin. Remember to return the foreskin to its proper location after inspection is complete. Look at the location of the urethral meatus and gently compress the glans between your gloved thumb and index finger which will open the urinary meatus to assess for any discharge.

Inspect the urethral meatus for any sign of irritation or drainage. If drainage is reported by the patient but not seen on inspection, you may gently squeeze to open the meatus to see if any discharge becomes visible. Milking the urethra may also result in visualization of discharge. Describe the amount and color of any discharge noted.

Inspect the scrotum for normal contour and any lesions present. Inspect the groin area for any signs of swelling or irritation. Patients who experience itching may demonstrate linear excoriations. Carefully inspect the excoriated area for lesions or nits.

Superficial inguinal nodes can be found just below the inguinal ligament, between the sartorius and adductor muscles in the groin. Deep inguinal nodes are located medial to the femoral vein. These lymph nodes drain the surface of the penis, the scrotum (in men), vulva (in women), perineum, buttocks, and lower abdominal wall.

Bladder fullness may cause discomfort in the suprapubic area. Gentle palpation of the suprapubic area may cause an increase in discomfort and result in an urge to urinate. A full bladder will feel somewhat like a water balloon. Percussion over a full bladder will produce a dull sound.

Palpation of the kidney can be achieved by deep palpation in the upper abdomen near the costal margins. The kidneys are located deep in the upper abdomen, protected from trauma. The right kidney is more readily palpated than the left kidney, since it is situated slightly lower in the abdomen.

Percussion on the back may cause pain in the kidney area in the setting of infection or kidney stones. Place your nondominant hand flat against the patient's back lateral to the vertebral column at the base of the ribs. This area is known as the costovertebral angle (CVA). Using the ulnar side of a closed fist (dominant hand), strike your nondominant hand. This percussion should not produce tenderness. Presence of CVA tenderness should be noted in the patient record. If the patient is experiencing flank area pain, percuss the opposite side first. Percussion of the nonaffected side may produce pain in the affected side. In this case, percussion of the affected side is not necessary as tenderness has already been determined.

The prostate can be assessed during a rectal examination. The posterior portion of the prostate can be palpated through the anterior rectal wall by an inserted index finger. Gloves should be worn for this examination. A small amount of water-soluble lubricant is applied to the index finger before the examination. Before the examination, the patient should be explained that they will feel pressure, but the examination will not cause pain.

Expected Findings

In a normal examination, this skin should be intact and you should not see any lesions, discharge, nits, or lice. You may note a whitish material (smegma) under the foreskin. The urethral meatus should be found slightly ventral to center in the glans.

The skin on the scrotum should appear to be slightly loose or wrinkled. The scrotum should be slightly lower on the left side as the left testis is positioned slightly lower than the right.

Normal lymph nodes are often not palpable. Use the finger pads (they are more sensitive) to palpate the area. If the nodes are palpable, they should be nontender, mobile, rubbery, and relatively small (<0.5 cm).

Under normal circumstances, the bladder is emptied regularly and not palpable unless there is a problem with emptying.

Deep palpation of the upper abdomen does not always result in being able to feel the kidney. The right kidney is the easier one to palpate as it is located somewhat lower in the abdomen. If the kidney is palpated, it should feel firm and smooth. Kidneys are more easily palpated in thin patients.

Percussion of the costovertebral area should not cause pain.

Palpation of the prostate should reveal a rubbery feel with a smooth surface on both lobes with a depressed median sulcus. Note any enlargement, nodules, or irregularity in shape.

Abnormal Findings

If you see any lesions, note the size, location, color, and any associated tenderness, induration, or discharge. Note the location of the urinary meatus. Hypospadias is a congenital condition where the urinary meatus is found on the ventral surface or underside of the penis. The penis may have a downward curvature during erection. Epispadias is a congenital condition where the urinary meatus is found on the top or side of the penis. The penis may be short, wide, and curved (see Figure 12-3). Urinary incontinence may occur.

Swelling within the scrotal area may be due to indirect hernias, hydroceles, or varicoceles. For patients with enlargement of the scrotal area due to hernia, bowel sounds may be auscultated within the scrotum. Hydroceles cause buildup of fluid within the scrotum and the scrotal area will transilluminate if a penlight is placed against the skin. This transillumination is due to the light traveling through the fluid-filled area. Varicoceles are due to varicose veins within the scrotum. This condition is more evident when the patient is standing up. Painful swelling may be due to testicular torsion, acute epididymitis, orchitis, or strangulated hernia. Pain on palpation of the posterolateral testicular area may be due to epididymitis.

If you notice inflammation of the glans, this may be due to balanitis.

Lymph nodes that are tender, fixed, hard, or enlarged are either due to reaction to infection or malignancy.

A full bladder has a slightly firm feeling on palpation, similar to a water balloon under the skin. The patient may experience discomfort or the sensation of the need to urinate when the bladder is palpated.

Kidney palpation should not reveal an uneven surface, nodules, or a hard area. CVA tenderness on percussion is found in patients with infection in or around the kidney or in those with renal stones.

Prostate enlargement may be due to normal changes of aging or the result of cancer. Note any nodules or irregularity in shape. Loss of the median sulcus is

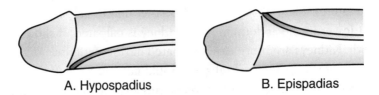

A. Hypospadius   B. Epispadias

FIGURE 12-3 • Illustration of hypospadias and epispadias.
(Reproduced with permission from LeBlond RF, DeGowin RL, Brown DD: *DeGowin's Diagnostic Examination*, 9th edition. New York, NY: McGraw-Hill; 2008. Figure 12-7 C&D.)

often due to enlargement of the gland. A gland that feels softer than normal, which is also called boggy, may be infected. A hard gland or nodule may be due to tumors or other disease.

Age-Related Changes

Pediatric

Normal developmental changes occur during puberty. There are five stages of puberty, often referred to as the Tanner stages. The Tanner Stage 1 is the pre-pubertal stage where physical sexual development has not yet begun, but hormonal activity is beginning. This change in hormonal activity typically occurs between the ages of 9 and 12 years. The Tanner Stage 2 is when the first visible signs of puberty occur, there is enlargement of the testicles and scrotum, and pubic hair begins to develop at the base of the penis. The beginning of the growth spurt occurs in this stage. During the Tanner Stage 3, the penis becomes longer (but not wider) and the testicles and scrotum continue to grow. Pubic hair becomes darker and coarser and starts to spread toward the legs. The voice starts to change, becoming deeper. The majority of the growth spurt occurs during the third stage. Ejaculation may occur at nighttime (wet dreams). During the Tanner Stage 4, the penis increases in width as well as length. The skin on the penis and scrotum becomes darker in color. Axillary hair develops, facial hair develops on the upper lip and chin, and pubic hair development is similar to that in an adult in appearance but covers less area. Acne is more common during this stage as the skin becomes oilier. Ejaculations occur, but not only at nighttime. During the Tanner Stage 5, the outer physical appearance is that of an adult.

Geriatric

Normal age-related changes can be expected as men age. There is a decrease in the amount of pubic hair. The glans becomes paler in color. The penis becomes smaller in length and thickness, more notable when the penis is erect. Older, overweight patients also have the added appearance of a shorter penis due to the presence of fat in the prepubic area. The testicles also become smaller in size with age. Some men develop scar tissue within the penis, which may be distributed unevenly. In this case, the penis becomes curved which may result in painful intercourse or may interfere with intercourse. There is a decrease in the sensitivity of the penis.

Cultural Considerations

Examination of the genital area may cause embarrassment for the patient. Certain cultures prefer that the examination be completed by a healthcare provider of the same gender.

The presence of hematuria and flank pain may be due to a parasitic infection known as schistosomiasis. This infection presents a notable public health issue outside of the US, particularly in Africa and the Middle East. Patients who are from these regions or those who have recently traveled to these areas are at risk for this type of infection.

CASE STUDY

Eddie is a 78-year-old man who experiences nocturia several times a night and has recently noted difficulty in initiating a urinary stream. The urinary stream is also less forceful than previously. He denies any burning sensation or dysuria.

REVIEW QUESTIONS

1. **Nocturia is best described as:**
   A. the need to urinate during the nighttime, which disrupts sleep.
   B. the sudden urge to urinate.
   C. urinating more frequently than is typical.
   D. discomfort of the urethra while urinating.

2. **On examination of the genital area, you note that the urethral opening is located on the ventral surface of the penis. This is correctly documented as:**
   A. hypospadias.
   B. epispadias.
   C. schistosomiasis.
   D. balanitis.

3. **Difficulty in initiating a urinary stream is described as:**
   A. urinary frequency.
   B. urgency.
   C. hesitancy.
   D. a feeling of bladder fullness despite having just emptied the bladder.

4. **Costovertebral angle (CVA) tenderness is typically due to:**
   A. kidney failure.
   B. hormonal changes of puberty.
   C. infection or kidney stones.
   D. excessive intake of water.

5. **Dysuria is best described as:**
   A. the presence of blood in the urine.
   B. discomfort associated with urination.
   C. anal discomfort experienced during urination.
   D. leakage of small amounts of urine from the urethra between episodes of urination.

6. **The patient is complaining of scrotal discomfort. On examination, the scrotal area appears swollen and transillumination is present. The healthcare provider suspects:**
   A. hydrocele.
   B. varicocele.
   C. epididymitis.
   D. hernia.

7. **The patient is admitted to the hospital and is being prepared for a surgical repair of a hernia. If there is scrotal enlargement due to the displacement of intestinal contents into the scrotal area, the expected finding is:**
   A. that the area will transilluminate.
   B. that the enlargement is more pronounced when the patient is standing.
   C. serous drainage over the affected area.
   D. bowel sounds that can be heard within the scrotum.

8. **The healthcare provider is reviewing the medical record of an adolescent male and see the notation of the Tanner Stage 4. TheTanner Stage 4 is:**
   A. the prepubertal stage where physical sexual development has not yet begun, but hormonal activity is beginning.
   B. when the first visible signs of puberty occur, there is enlargement of the testicles and scrotum and pubic hair begins to grow at the base of the penis. The beginning of the growth spurt also occurs in this stage.
   C. when the penis becomes longer, but not wider, and the testicles and scrotum continue to grow. Pubic hair becomes darker and coarser and starts to spread toward the legs. The voice starts to deepen. The majority of the growth spurt occurs during the third stage. Ejaculation may occur at nighttime (wet dreams).
   D. when the penis increases in width and length and the skin on the penis and scrotum becomes darker in color. Axillary and facial hair develops, and pubic hair is similar to an adult in appearance, but covers less area. Acne is also more common during this stage.

9. **Which of the following would be expected findings on palpation of a distended bladder?**

   A. It will feel slightly firm on palpation.
   B. The patient may experience discomfort.
   C. The patient may experience a feeling that they need to urinate.
   D. All of the above.

10. **Which of the following would be considered an *abnormal* finding on palpation of the posterior aspect of the prostate gland?**

   A. The presence of a median sulcus.
   B. A firm, regular surface.
   C. A boggy or soft surface.
   D. Even symmetry.

ANSWERS

1. A.
   B. Urgency is the sudden need to urinate.
   C. Frequency is urinating more often than is typical.
   D. Dysuria is urethral discomfort during urinating.

2. A.
   B. Epispadias is a congenital condition where the urinary meatus is found on the top or side of the penis.
   C. Schistosomiasis is a parasitic infection.
   D. Balanitis is inflammation of the glans of the penis.

3. C.
   A. Urinary frequency is the need to urinate more often.
   B. Urgency is the need the need to urinate immediately.
   D. The feeling of bladder fullness despite having just emptied the bladder can occur with an enlarged prostate.

4. C.
   A. Kidney failure should not result in pain on percussion.
   B. Hormonal changes of puberty should not result in pain on percussion.
   D. Excessive intake of water may result in electrolyte changes but should not result in pain on percussion.

5. B.

   A. The presence of blood in the urine is hematuria.

   C. Anal discomfort experienced during urination is an abnormal symptom and may be due to infection or inflammation of the prostate gland.

   D. Leakage of small amounts of urine from the urethra between episodes of urination can occur with an enlarged prostate and is typically referred to as dribbling.

6. A.

   B. Varicocele occurs with enlarged, tortuous veins within the scrotum.

   C. Epididymitis is a painful inflammation where the epididymis attaches to the testicle.

   D. Hernia may displace bowel contents into the scrotal area, but will not transilluminate.

7. D.

   A. Hydroceles will transilluminate.

   B. The scrotal enlargement may be more pronounced when the patient is standing when a varicocele is present.

   C. There should not be any drainage.

8. D.

   A. The stage with the beginning of hormonal activity and a prepubertal appearance is Tanner Stage 1.

   B. The first visible signs of puberty occur and beginning of a growth spurt occur in Tanner Stage 2.

   C. The penis lengthens, scrotum and testicles grow, pubic hair becomes darker and coarser in Tanner Stage 3.

9. D. A distended bladder should feel slightly firm and may cause the patient to feel discomfort or the urge to urinate.

10. C. The presence of a median sulcus, a firm, regular surface and even symmetry are expected findings.

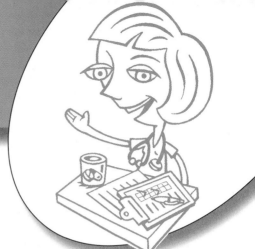

chapter 13

Assessment of the Female Reproductive System

LEARNING OBJECTIVES

After reviewing this chapter, the learner will be able to:

1. Identify important anatomic landmarks of the gynecologic system and breast.
2. Discuss the appropriate information to gather during an interview.
3. Demonstrate a physical assessment of the gynecologic system and breast.
4. List normal physical assessment findings.
5. Describe abnormal physical assessment findings.
6. Discuss the age-related differences related to the gynecologic system and breast.

KEYWORDS

Adipose tissue

Axillary lymph nodes

Bartholin cyst

Colostrum

Fundus

Human papillomavirus (HPV)

Mammary ridge

Menorrhagia

Mons pubis

Perineum

Introduction

Women's health involves gynecology and breast health. Disorders involving the female reproductive tract or breast can have a significant effect on the patient. Either of these may be very distressing to the patient. Patients and caregivers may feel uncomfortable in discussing issues involving the women's health. It is important to make the patient feel at ease in discussing all health-related topics. Healthcare providers may need to overcome their own discomfort in discussing what may be sensitive topics.

Review of Anatomy and Physiology

Female reproductive organs are located within the pelvic cavity. The uterus is a hollow organ and commonly described as being pear shaped (see Figure 13-1). In an adult, it is approximately 6 cm long. The cervix is located at the base of the uterus. The fallopian tubes are located bilaterally and are attached to the fundus (upper area) of the uterus. The adult fallopian tubes are about 10 cm long. The ovaries are oval in shape and located near the open ends of the fallopian tubes.

There is an area of adipose tissue over the symphysis pubis, which protects the area from trauma. It is called the mons pubis (see Figure 13-2). The labia majora are external skin folds, which are located between the mons pubis and the perineal area. The labia minora are smaller folds of skin that are located between the labia majora. The glans clitoris comprises erectile tissue and is located at the anterior area where the labia minora meet. The vestibule is the opening located between the labia minora. The vaginal introitus (opening) and urethral meatus are located within the vestibule. The adult vagina is about 2-4 inches in length. The walls of the vagina contain rugae (a corrugated surface—think of folds in the mucosa). There is a healthy balance of bacteria

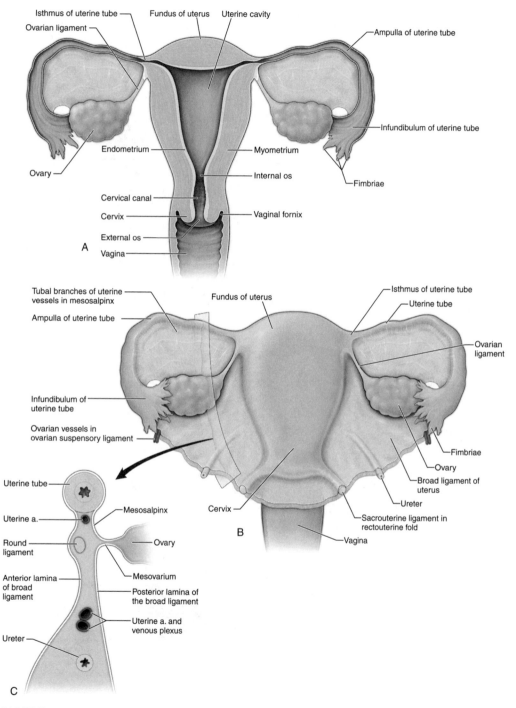

FIGURE 13-1 • Uterus and uterine tubes.
(Reproduced with permission from Morton DA, Foreman KB, Albertine KH: *The Big Picture: Gross Anatomy*. New York, NY: McGraw-Hill; 2011. Figure 14-1.)

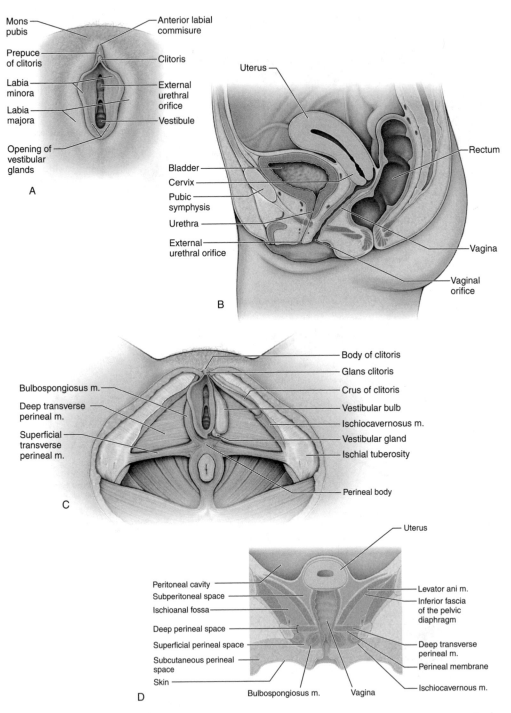

FIGURE 13-2 • Female reproductive anatomy.
(Reproduced with permission from Morton DA, Foreman KB, Albertine KH: *The Big Picture: Gross Anatomy.* New York, NY: McGraw-Hill; 2011. Figure 14-2.)

and yeast present within the vagina. Vaginal moisture is maintained by the presence of mucus. The amount, consistency, and chemical composition vary during the menstrual cycle. The mucus becomes more slippery during ovulation. The hymen is a delicate membranous tissue that is located at the vaginal introitus. The perineum is the area between the vagina and the anus.

There is a significant variability in breast size among individuals, but the basic anatomic structures of the adult breast remain the same. Breast tissue may extend from the sternal border to the anterior axillary line. A portion of breast tissue is located in the upper, outer area, toward the axilla. This extended area is the Tail of Spence. It is important to examine this area as breast cancer can occur in this area. The breast tissue lies on top of the pectoral muscle on the chest wall, above the ribcage. Each breast contains adipose tissue and has multiple lobes that are arranged alongside each other around the breast, like the spokes on a wheel. Within the lobes, smaller structures called lobules have small bulbs on the end where milk is produced. There are a multitude of ducts that connect these structures and allow for the passage of milk. These ducts all lead to the nipple. The adipose tissue fills the space between the lobes, lobules, and ducts (see Figure 13-3). A pigmented areola surrounds the nipple. The mammary ridge or crease is the posterior border of the breast. It is a palpable ridge of tissue that helps support the breast.

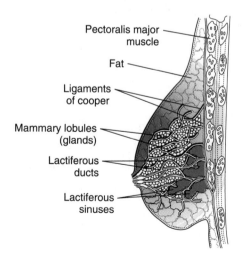

FIGURE 13-3 • Cross section of breast.
(Reproduced with permission from DeCherney AH, Nathan L, Laufer N et al: *Current Diagnosis & Treatment: Obstetrics & Gynecology*, 11th edition. New York, NY: McGraw-Hill; 2012. Figure 5-1.)

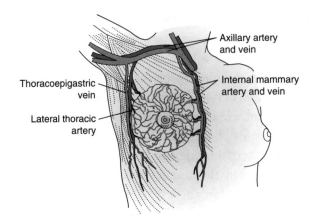

FIGURE 13-4 • Vascular supply of breast.
(Reproduced with permission from DeCherney AH, Nathan L, Laufer N et al: *Current Diagnosis & Treatment: Obstetrics & Gynecology*, 11th edition. New York, NY: McGraw-Hill; 2012. Figure 5-2.)

Lymphatic vessels within the breast drain into the lymph nodes found under the arm (axillary), above the clavicle (supraclavicular) and within the chest. The axillary lymph nodes are divided into three levels. Level I (low-level) nodes are found to the side of the pectoralis minor muscle. The Level II (mid-level) nodes are behind or under the pectoralis minor muscle. Level III (high-level) nodes are medial and superior to the pectoralis minor muscle. Axillary lymph nodes include the pectoral (anterior), brachial (lateral), sub-scapular (posterior), central and subscapular (medial) chains (see Figures 13-4 and 13-5). Picture the axillary area as an upside down box. This image will help you to palpate all sides of the "box."

Subjective Information

Interview

Both patients and healthcare providers may experience some discomfort in discussing personal details related to sexual function, reproduction, and/or breast conditions. Care should be taken to enhance the patient's comfort in discussing these topics.

Review of Systems (ROS)

Gynecologic

It is important to determine the date of the last menstrual period (LMP) for women of childbearing age. This is the day of onset of menses. Some women

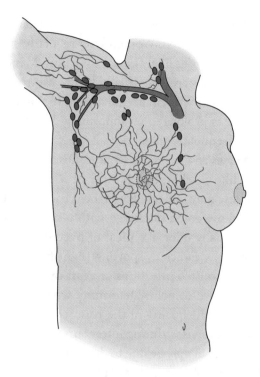

FIGURE 13-5 • Lymph nodes for breast area.
(Reproduced with permission from DeCherney AH, Nathan L, Laufer N et al: *Current Diagnosis & Treatment: Obstetrics & Gynecology*, 11th edition. New York, NY: McGraw-Hill; 2012. Figure 5-3.)

find it easier to determine the date when they look at a calendar. For women who are menopausal the answer may be an age, rather than an exact date. Ask the menopausal patient if they experienced any associated symptoms, such as hot flashes or night sweats. Ask about any spotting or bleeding since their last period. Spotting or bleeding in a menopausal woman may indicate serious disease. Ask about any hormone replacement therapy. Long term use of combination (estrogen-progestin) hormonal therapy has been linked to an increased risk of cardiovascular disease (such as heart attack and stroke), breast cancer, and blood clot formation.

A more thorough menstrual history should be completed for women of childbearing age, or in those having gynecologic complaints. Ask how old the patient was at menarche (onset of menses). Find out how often the woman menstruates. Most women menstruate about the same time each month, but there is a normal variation of 25-35 days between cycles. Ask how many days the bleeding lasts. Ask if the bleeding is light, moderate, or heavy. Not all women are sure which of those options applies (since they have nothing to compare with), so it may be better to ask how many sanitary pads or tampons are used each day, and what absorbency is used. Women who regularly stain their clothes or experience clots during menses likely have heavy flow. Menorrhagia is the term used when menstrual cycles are abnormally heavy. Metrorrhagia is used when menstrual cycles that occur with an irregular pattern. Menometrorrhagia is the term used when there is prolonged or abnormally heavy bleeding that occurs irregularly and more frequently than normal.

Ask if she experiences any vaginal discharge. Discharge may signal infection. Thick, white, curd-like discharge is typical of a candida (yeast) infection. Cloudy white or yellow may indicate gonorrhea. Trichomoniasis infection typically has a frothy, yellow-green discharge with a noticeable odor. A white to gray discharge with a fishy odor is typical of bacterial vaginosis. A bloody or brown discharge typically indicates spotting (light bleeding). Ask if there is a history of sexually transmitted infections or yeast infection.

Ask about the presence of pain. Determine where the pain is felt (lower abdomen, vagina, labia), the quality of the pain (cramping, sharp, dull, or aching), the timing (during menses, during intercourse), and any associated symptoms (discharge, fever). Pain may be due to dysmenorrhea (cramping discomfort associated with the onset of menses in some women), infection (pelvic inflammatory disease or pelvic inflammatory disease [PID]), or ovarian cyst. Women who have a complaint of abdominal pain should have a gynecologic evaluation to rule out serious health problems, such as ectopic pregnancy, ruptured ovarian cysts, or PID.

Ask the patient about the use of birth control. Barrier methods can be effective in preventing infections that are transmitted through exchange of body fluids (hepatitis, human immunodeficiency virus [HIV], sexually transmitted diseases) if used consistently and properly. Hormonal methods of birth control are more effective at preventing pregnancy when used appropriately. Both barrier methods and hormonal methods are designed to prevent conception. Intrauterine devices (IUDs) are implanted and create an inhospitable environment for implantation of a fertilized ovum within the uterus. Some IUDs also release a hormone that thickens the cervical mucus and causes the lining of the uterus to be thinner than usual. It is very important for some patients to know whether the method of birth control they are considering will prevent conception. Tubal ligation is a common surgical sterilization for women. In this procedure, the fallopian tubes are cut or sealed to prevent sperm from meeting an ovum.

Ask about pregnancy. Most facilities use either GPA (gravida/para/abortus) or TPAL (term/premature/abortion/living) method of recording the obstetric history of the patient. Gravida is the term used for the number of times the woman has been pregnant, regardless of the outcome of the pregnancy. Para refers to the number of deliveries. Abortus/abortion refers to spontaneous abortion (miscarriage) or elective abortion before 20 weeks gestation. If the patient is pregnant for the first time, she would be gravida 1, para 0, abortus 0. Term refers to the number of pregnancies delivered at 38 weeks gestational age or greater. Premature refers to the number of pregnancies delivered before 38 weeks gestation. Living refers to the number of living children that the patient has delivered.

Breast

Ask the patient about any changes in the breast. The presence of pain may occur with infection or the presence of cysts. Ask the patient if they perform self-breast examinations. If so, how often are they performed? The best time for breast examinations is 1 week after the start of the menstrual cycle. If the woman does not perform breast examinations, ask if she knows how. A surprising number of women have never been taught how to do this.

Ask about any masses or lumps. This may have been discovered during breast self-examination or found incidentally during a shower. Ask about any visible changes. Redness or a rash on the skin may indicate infection. Skin with a swollen, pitted surface (referred to as *peau d'orange*) may be associated with breast cancer. Ask about the appearance of the nipple. Some women normally have inverted (inward) nipples. A woman who suddenly develops an inverted nipple should have a clinical breast examination to further evaluate this change. Dimpling of the skin on the breast could signify that there is pulling on the skin from inside the breast.

Ask about the presence of any discharge from the nipple. Women who are in the later part of pregnancy may note fluid leaking from the nipple. This may be clear or yellowish and is referred to as colostrum. Women who are breast-feeding may experience a discharge of milk from the breast in response to their baby crying, direct stimulation of the breast, or if it is time to feed their baby. Nipple discharge is not a normal finding in a woman who is not pregnant or breastfeeding. If discharge is present, ask whether it occurs unilaterally or bilaterally. The discharge may be due to a benign or cancerous breast condition or a systemic disorder (such as hormonal imbalance, trauma, or certain medications). Ask the patient to describe the discharge. Bloody discharge should be further evaluated as it can sometimes occur with breast cancer. Disorders that increase the prolactin level can result in galactorrhea (milky discharge from the breast).

Risk Factors Related to the System

Gynecologic

Sexually transmitted infections may be asymptomatic and can cause problems with fertility.

There are multiple (over 150) strains of human papillomavirus (HPV), but only about 40 that affect the genital and anal areas. Strains 16 and 18 have been linked to cervical cancer. It is also associated with vulvar, vaginal, penile, anal, and oropharyngeal cancers. HPV is the most common sexually transmitted infection and can be transmitted during vaginal, anal, or oral sex, or during skin to skin contact such as genital to genital contact without intercourse.

Risks for cervical cancer include HPV infection, smoking, multiple pregnancies, and long-term oral contraceptive use.

Breast

Breast cancer risk factors include being female, advancing age, genetics, family history, personal history of breast cancer, race, certain breast conditions, and menstrual history.

BRCA1 and *BRCA2* are genetic mutations linked to breast cancer that may be inherited from either parent. The US women of Ashkenazi Jewish descent have a greater incidence of *BRCA* mutations. Genetic testing can identify the presence of these mutations. Careful counseling of patients is needed to weigh the benefit versus the risk of knowing the test result for each individual patient.

Patients who have a first-degree relative (mother, sister, or daughter) with breast cancer have about twice the risk of developing breast cancer compared with those without a first-degree relative with breast cancer. An increased number of first-degree relatives with breast cancer significantly increase the risk of developing breast cancer. Family history of breast cancer is present in up to 15% of women with breast cancer.

Caucasian women are slightly more likely than other ethnicities to develop breast cancer overall. Breast cancer that develops in a premenopausal woman is more common in African American women. There is a lower risk of developing breast cancer in Asian, Hispanic, or Native American women.

There are many conditions that affect the breast, which are benign. The presence of some of these conditions does actually increase the risk of developing breast cancer. There is a mild increase in the risk of developing breast cancer with fibroadenoma or ductal hyperplasia without atypia. There is a more significantly increased risk of developing breast cancer in patients with atypical ductal hyperplasia or atypical lobar hyperplasia. Patients with lobular carcinoma *in situ* (LCIS—cancerous cells growing only within the lobules where milk is produced, and there is no spread found beyond the lobule walls) have a significant increase in risk of developing breast cancer.

Women who had an early menarche (onset of menses) and late menopause (cessation of menses) have an increased risk of developing breast cancer.

Diethylstilbestrol (DES) is a medication that was given to pregnant women during the middle of the 20th century. Women who took the medication themselves, or who were exposed *in utero* (during pregnancy) have a slight increase in the risk of developing breast cancer.

The hereditary breast and ovarian cancer (HBOC) syndrome is a concern for patients who have a family history of early (before the age of 50 years) onset of breast cancer, both breast and ovarian cancers, bilateral cancers (occurring in both breasts or both ovaries), prostate cancer, male family members with breast cancer, or if the patients are of Ashkenazi Jewish, Icelandic, Dutch, or Swedish ancestry. The HBOC syndrome has an autosomal dominant genetic pattern. The altered gene can be transmitted by either parent. An abnormal or mutated gene will be transmitted from parent to child and there needs to be a second genetic mutation for cancer to develop.

The majority of breast cancers are not hereditary, but the risk of developing breast cancer when the genes are present can be as high as 80%. Risk for breast, ovarian, prostate, stomach, laryngeal cancers, and melanoma is increased with the presence of *BRCA1* or *BRCA2*.

Risk Evaluation

Gynecologic

The HPV vaccine is recommended for preteen-aged males and females, between the ages of 11 and 12 years during a routine pediatric visit. It is approved for use between the age of 9 years and up to the age of 26 years in women and up to the age of 21 years in men. It is recommended for adolescents and young adults who have not previously received the vaccine. It is administered in a series of three injections over a period of 6 months.

Cervical cancer screening is routinely done with a Papanicolaou test, more commonly called a Pap test or Pap smear. It is recommended for women between the ages of 21 and 65 years to check for the presence of abnormal cervical cells. HPV screening is recommended for women over 30 years of age. Women with normal Pap tests and HPV screenings can be tested every 3 years. Women over the age of 65 years with a history of only normal Pap tests can stop Pap tests after consulting with their healthcare provider.

Breast

Monthly self-breast examination is no longer recommended as it does not significantly increase the chance of the patient discovering changes related to breast cancer. It is still an option for assessment, and women who perform the examination regularly are more familiar with the look and feel of their breasts and are more readily able to identify changes.

Clinical breast examinations are performed by physicians, nurse practitioners, physician assistants, and nurses. They are recommended every 3 years for women aged 20-39 years and annually starting at the age of 40 years.

Annual mammograms are recommended for women beginning at the age of 40 years. Annual screening mammograms should continue as long as the patient is in good health otherwise.

Objective Information

Equipment Needed

Light source, gloves, drape for privacy, and speculum.

Assessment Techniques

Inspection, palpation.

Physical Examination

Gynecologic

Instruct the patient not to douche, have sexual intercourse, use birth control cream, jelly or foam, vaginal creams or medications, or use a tampon for 1-2 days before having a Pap test. It is preferred to complete the examination when the woman is not menstruating. The patient should undress and wear a disposable gown, open in the front. Provide a drape for privacy. The patient should lie down on the examination table. Assist the patient into a lithotomy position, placing her heels in the footrests. Instruct the patient to slide down until she feels her buttocks just past the edge of the table. There should be a pillow for her head.

Inspect the mons pubis, labia, and perineum. Warn the patient that she will feel your hand, and then separate the labia to inspect the labia minora, clitoris, urethral meatus, and vaginal opening.

Disposable specula are most commonly used. Select a size (small, medium, or large) that is appropriate to the patient. Moisten the specula with warm water to ease insertion. Warn the patient that you are about to insert the speculum. Gently press the index finger of your nondominant hand with mild pressure against the posterior area of the vaginal introitus. Gently insert the closed speculum on an angle (approximately 25 degrees off of vertical) with a downward and backward motion over your index finger. As you insert the speculum, gently rotate it to horizontal. The downward pressure is needed to avoid undue trauma to the urethra or clitoris. Avoid pulling on any pubic hair or pinching the labia. Once the speculum is completely inserted, gently open the blades. You should see the cervix within the opening created. If you do not see the cervix, gently pull back the speculum slightly and reinsert with a more anterior angle. Once the cervix is visualized, lock the speculum. If there is a lot of cervical mucus, gently wipe it away with large cotton swabs. Note the appearance of the cervix, including position, characteristics of the surface, or discharge from the cervical os. Any necessary specimens are obtained at this time.

Unlock the speculum and maintain the open position of the blades. Slowly withdraw the speculum and note the appearance of the vaginal mucosa. Let the speculum slowly close as it is withdrawn, taking care not to pinch the delicate tissue.

Breast

Inspect the breasts while the patient is comfortably seated on an examination table with her arms at her sides. Ask her to raise her arms over her head, then put her hands on her hips and press down with her hands, then lean forward with her chest parallel to the floor. Inspect the breasts from each position, noting shape, symmetry, skin appearance, any dimpling, or retractions.

Assist the patient to recline on the examination table. Remember to support the lower legs (you may need to pull out the leg rest on some tables) and give her a pillow for her head. Ask the patient to raise the arm on the side you are about to examine over her head while lying down comfortably. Drape the opposite side for privacy. Let the patient know that you are about to touch her as part of the breast examination. Using the finger pads of three fingers (index, middle, and ring fingers) of your dominant hand, begin to palpate the breast tissue using a circular motion. Use a systematic approach (horizontal, vertical, or circular) until the entire area is examined. When moving your fingers, slightly overlap the area that was just examined. Be sure to assess the Tail of Spence. When you have completed one breast examination, cover the patient and move to the other side of the patient. Have the patient raise the other arm and uncover the breast to be examined, leaving the other side of the patient covered for privacy. Complete the examination on the other side.

Assess the axillary lymph nodes after you have examined the breasts. Assist the patient to comfortably sit with her arms at her side. Gently move one arm away from her body and support the weight of the arm. Use your gloved finger pads pressing toward the patient's neck to palpate the medial nodes, press toward the front of the patient to assess the anterior nodes, press toward the patient's back to assess the posterior nodes and toward the patient's arm to assess the lateral nodes of the axilla. Palpate posterior to the pectoral muscle and anterior to the lateral border of the scapula.

Expected Findings

Gynecologic

The cervix should be round with an even surface. The cervical os (opening) should be small and round in a nulliparous woman, and a short, curved line (like a smile) in a parous woman. The vaginal mucosa should be pink and moist. Note the rugae (folds) on the vaginal walls.

Breast

The breast tissue comprises ducts, lobules, and fatty tissue. It typically feels uneven and lumpy. You may be able to palpate milk ducts and supporting structures in older women, and these have a somewhat cord-like feel.

You often do not palpate any axillary nodes.

Abnormal Findings

Gynecologic

Inflammation, discharge, swelling, ulcerations, or nodules are abnormal and warrant further evaluation. If there is posterior (about 4 o'clock and 8 o'clock positions) labial swelling, you should assess for the presence of a Bartholin cyst. You should gently palpate the area between your thumb and forefinger. This may be painful for the patient. It is common to culture the discharge from this area.

An uneven surface, polyps, nodules, or discharge within the cervical os are considered abnormal. Friability (bleeding when touching the cervix) is not expected. During pregnancy, however, the cervix may be friable.

Inflammation, discharge, masses, or ulcerations on the vaginal walls are abnormal and warrant further investigation.

Breast

Asymmetry, nipple retraction (if new for the patient), or skin changes (such as dimpling or *peau d'orange*) are abnormal.

Nipple discharge is abnormal unless the patient is in the later stages of pregnancy or is breastfeeding.

Discrete masses or nodes in the axillary area are likely abnormal. Note the firmness (hard versus rubbery), size, location, mobility (mobile or fixed), pain on palpation (nontender versus tender). Adenopathy may be due to infection.

Age-Related Changes

Pediatric

The hormonal changes associated with puberty result in sexual maturation and the development of secondary sexual characteristics. Development of the breast tissue and pubic hair occur before the onset of menstruation (menarche). Menarche occurs at different ages, depending on hormonal activity, but the average age is 12 years. Ovulation typically begins after the onset of menstruation, and may take 1-2 years to become regular. Axillary hair development commonly occurs after menstruation begins. Tanner staging is a commonly used system for describing the stages of puberty (see Figure 13-6).

Gynecologic

Tanner Stage 1 is preadolescent development. Pubic hair is vellus and in the same quantity as other areas of the body. (Fig. 13-6, P1)

Tanner Stage 2 has the development of a few long, straight (or slightly curled), pigmented hair along the labia. (Fig 13-6, P2)

Tanner Stage 3 has an increase in the amount of darker, curlier, coarse pubic hair that spreads slightly higher. (Fig. 13-6, P3)

Tanner Stage 4 has a greater increase in the amount of pubic hair that has the characteristics of adult pubic hair, but of a lesser distribution. There is no spread to the thigh area. (Fig. 13-6, P4)

Tanner Stage 5 the pubic hair is adult in appearance and distribution, appearing as an inverse triangle. There may be a spread to the medial thigh area. (Fig 13-6, P5)

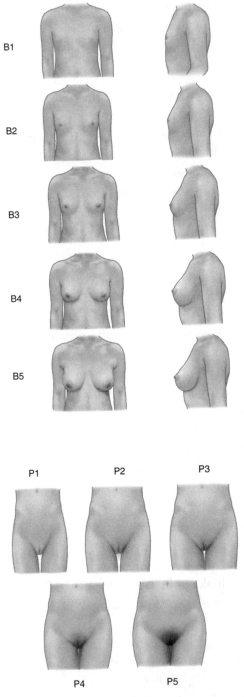

FIGURE 13-6 • The Tanner stages of female breast and pubic hair development. (Reproduced with permission from Hoffman BL, Schorge JO, Schaffer JI et al: *Williams Gynecology*, 2nd edition. New York, NY: McGraw-Hill; 2012. Figure 14-3.)

Breast

Tanner Stage 1 is preadolescent. There is elevation of the nipple only. (Fig. 13-6, B1)

Tanner Stage 2 is referred to as breast budding. There is elevation of the breast and nipple as a small mound with an increase in the diameter of the areolae. (Fig. 13-6, B2)

Tanner Stage 3 has further enlargement of the breast and areolae, without any separation in contour. (Fig. 13-6, B3)

Tanner Stage 4 shows further enlargement of the breast tissue with a secondary mound formed by the elevation of the areolae and nipples. (Fig. 13-6, B4)

Tanner Stage 5 is adult breast appearance. (Fig. 13-6, B5)

Geriatric

Gynecologic

Menopause is the complete cessation of menses. For a while before menopause, the woman may experience periods that are irregular (longer or shorter than usual, erratic occurrence, or changes in amount of flow). This time is referred to as perimenopause. Menopause typically occurs at about the age of 50 years. The normal age range for menopause is 45-55 years. Menopause may be accompanied by moodiness, hot flashes, headaches, insomnia, or difficulty with short-term memory. Some women experience a decrease in libido (sex drive). Women are considered menopausal when they have had no menstrual bleeding or spotting for one full year. Vaginal bleeding after menopause is considered abnormal and needs further evaluation. There may be prolapse of the uterus or bladder due to loss of muscle tone.

The vaginal area becomes drier and there is some normal tissue atrophy (thinning) as women age and the rugae become less prominent. There is less elasticity of the vaginal musculature. Hormonal changes of aging may result in vaginal dryness that may cause irritation (atrophic vaginitis). Some women experience mild irritation with urination due to dryness. It is important to determine the cause of the irritation, as both urinary tract infections and dryness may be causative. The labia may also undergo atrophy (shrink). The pubic hair may become gray and sparser with aging.

Breast

The breasts are less full and there is some sagging that occurs as the supporting structures become more lax. Nipple size decreases and there is less response to stimulation. Milk-producing glands are replaced with fat.

Cultural Considerations

Some women may be accompanied by family members to gynecologic visits. In some cultures, family members (often men—the patient's husband or father) may be considered as the decision maker for the patient. Other patients may be concerned over being undressed in front of a healthcare provider (who is a stranger to the patient). Respect for the patient's wishes for modesty must be considered. Developmental differences may be the result of altered nutritional intake or poverty (a significant association between health disparity and poverty exists).

CASE STUDY

Amy is a 25-year-old woman who is scheduled for a routine gynecologic examination today. She has been pregnant twice and has a 2-year-old daughter and an 8-month-old son at home. She denies any history of sexually transmitted disease and has no current complaints.

REVIEW QUESTIONS

1. **If you were documenting Amy's obstetrical history using the GPA method, you would correctly note:**
   A. G 2 P 2 A 0.
   B. G 2 P 2 A 2.
   C. G 2 P 2 years, 8 months A 0.
   D. G 2 P 1 girl 1 boy A 1.

2. **Human papillomavirus (HPV) vaccine is recommended for females:**
   A. in early childhood, before they start school.
   B. between the ages of 11 and 26 years.
   C. during childbearing years, between the ages of 16 and 40 years.
   D. after menopause.

3. **Papanicolaou (or Pap) tests are recommended:**
   A. between the ages of 21 and 65 years.
   B. within 1 year of the onset of sexual activity.
   C. once the woman reaches Tanner Stage 2.
   D. starting at the age of 18 years.

4. **Risk for developing breast cancer is increased with:**

   A. the presence of *BRCA1* or *BRCA2* genetic mutation.
   B. having a first-degree relative with breast cancer.
   C. having a personal history of atypical ductal hyperplasia.
   D. having an early menarche and a late menopause.
   E. all of the above.

5. **Women who have had multiple normal Pap tests and are over the age of 30 years should have (*select all that apply*):**

   A. HPV screening.
   B. Pap tests every 3 years.
   C. annual Pap tests and HPV screening as long as they are sexually active.
   D. three doses of HPV vaccine.

6. **Perimenopause refers to the time:**

   A. between menarche and menopause.
   B. between onset of menses and regulation of ovulation.
   C. after menses has ceased for 1 year or more.
   D. before menopause when the menstrual cycle become erratic.

7. **The average age of onset of menses is at the age of:**

   A. 10 years.
   B. 12 years.
   C. 14 years.
   D. 16 years.

8. **Galactorrhea may occur due to:**

   A. heavy menstrual flow.
   B. decreased progesterone levels.
   C. increased prolactin levels.
   D. increased estrogen levels.

9. **Menorrhagia is a term that is best described as:**

   A. normal menstrual flow.
   B. menstrual cycles that occur on an irregular basis.
   C. prolonged or abnormally heavy bleeding that occurs more frequently than normal.
   D. menstrual cycles that are abnormally heavy.

10. **Which of the following sexually transmitted infections has been linked to cervical cancer?**

    A. Gonorrhea
    B. Chlamydia
    C. HPV
    D. Herpes

ANSWERS

1. A. She has had two pregnancies (G 2) and two deliveries (P 2) and no other pregnancies (A 0). Gravida is the number of pregnancies, para is the number of deliveries, and abortus is the number of spontaneous and elective abortions.

2. B. An HPV vaccine is approved for females between the ages of 9 and 26 years.

3. A. The Papanicolaou test is recommended between the ages of 21 and 65 years.

4. E. The presence of *BRCA1* or *BRCA2* genetic mutation, having a first-degree relative with breast cancer, having a personal history of atypical ductal hyperplasia, and having an early menarche and a late menopause all increase the risk for developing breast cancer.

5. A and B. Women who have had multiple normal Pap tests and are over the age of 30 years should have HPV screening and Pap tests every 3 years.

6. D. Perimenopause is the time before menopause when the menstrual cycle becomes erratic.

7. B. Twelve years of age is the average onset of menses.

8. C. Galactorrhea is a milky discharge from the breast and is often associated with elevated prolactin levels.

9. D. Menorrhagia refers to menstrual cycles that are abnormally heavy.

10. C. Human papillomavirus (HPV) has been linked to cervical cancer.

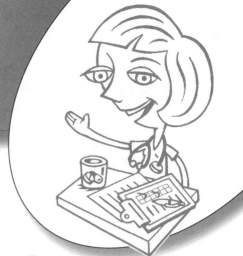

Assessment of the Pregnant Patient

After reviewing this chapter, the learner will be able to:

❶ Identify important anatomic landmarks of the pregnant woman.

❷ Discuss the appropriate information to gather during an interview.

❸ Demonstrate a physical assessment of the pregnant woman.

❹ List normal physical assessment findings.

❺ Describe abnormal physical assessment findings.

❻ Discuss the age-related differences related to the pregnant woman.

KEYWORDS

Chloasma
Human chorionic gonadotropin
(hCG)
Human placental lactogen (hPL)
Linea nigra
Lordosis

Multigravida
Preeclampsia
Preterm labor
Primigravida
Striae

Introduction

Some patients will seek healthcare because they are pregnant, whereas others will seek care for some other reason while they are pregnant. Conduction of health assessment during pregnancy is similar to the examination of the non-pregnant woman. The healthcare professional conducting the assessment must be aware of the effects that pregnancy has on the body and be able to differentiate between expected and unexpected changes.

Review of Anatomy and Physiology

A normal pregnancy usually lasts approximately 40 weeks. Pregnancy is divided into three trimesters. The first trimester is considered from Weeks 1 to 12. The second trimester is from Weeks 13 to 27, and the third trimester is from Weeks 28 to 40. A woman pregnant for the first time is referred to as a primigravida. A woman who has been pregnant more than once is a multigravida.

Pregnancy causes many physical changes in the woman. These changes are a result of both the increase in hormone production and the effects of the enlarged uterus and growing baby on the maternal physiologic functioning. One of the first signs of pregnancy is the absence of menstruation. Breast tenderness, fatigue, and mild, intermittent nausea (morning sickness) are fairly common during the early stages of pregnancy.

During pregnancy the placenta produces the hormones estrogen, progesterone, and human placental lactogen (hPL) (see Figure 14-1). Human chorionic gonadotropin (hCG) is also produced by the placenta. A pregnancy test detects the presence of hCG. The hCG levels can be detected in the mother's bloodstream before it can be detected in the urine. The hormones released by the

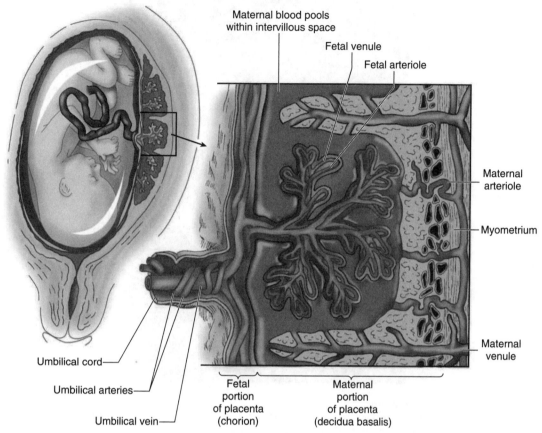

FIGURE 14-1 • The placenta.
(Reproduced with permission from Butterworth JF, Mackey DC, Wasnick JD: *Morgan & Mikhail's Clinical Anesthesiology*, 5th edition. New York, NY: McGraw-Hill; 2013. Figure 40-2.)

placenta are responsible for many of the physiologic changes that occur during the 9 months. The breasts enlarge and the nipples become darker as a result of estrogen production. The skin will have a change of pigmentation as a result of estrogen and progesterone production. It is common for the woman to develop a dark line of pigmentation from the pubic area to the upper abdomen. This line is called the linea nigra. The face may develop areas of increased pigmentation on the forehead, cheeks, and nose. This is known as chloasma (see Figure 14-2). Striae or stretch marks may develop on the abdomen and breasts. These initially appear as reddish brown lines. After the pregnancy they may change color to silvery white.

As the uterus enlarges during pregnancy, there is increased sensation of pressure on the adjacent organs. Different areas of the body are affected as the

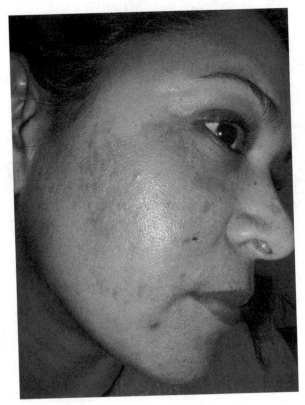

FIGURE 14-2 • Chloasma.
(Reproduced with permission from Usatine RP, Smith MA, Mayeaux EJ Jr, et al: *The Color Atlas of Family Medicine*. New York, NY: McGraw-Hill; 2009. Figure 4-3.)

pregnancy progresses. For example, the woman may complain of lower abdominal pressure in the first trimester of pregnancy due to the uterine pressure on the bladder. Increased frequency in urination is common in the first trimester. In the second trimester, as the uterus rises higher in the abdomen this pressure is relieved. In the third trimester, the fetus begins to descend into the pelvis and the sensation of lower abdominal pressure returns. In the third trimester, the growing baby results in a decreased space in the upper abdomen. This often causes symptoms such as shortness of breath or heartburn. The weight of the enlarged uterus and baby cause an increased strain on the muscles of the back, which in turn will increase complaints of back pain. The increased abdominal area weight in an advanced pregnancy alters the center of gravity for the expectant mother and results in a wider stance and lordosis (increased curvature of the lumbar area of the back). As physical changes and discomfort are more evident as the pregnancy progresses, some women note difficulty in sleeping.

Subjective Information

Interview

The date of the last menstrual period should be obtained. It should be noted if and where the woman has received prenatal care. The woman should be interviewed to determine if she has any complaints or problems associated with the pregnancy. It is important to document any complaints of pain, vaginal bleeding, or leakage of fluid. The healthcare provider should ask at every visit if the woman feels fetal movement.

Review of Systems (ROS)

The ROS is the same as for all adult health assessment.

Risk Evaluation

The healthcare provider needs to assess for preeclampsia and preterm labor when performing a health assessment on a pregnant woman. These are conditions that can affect the health of the mother and fetus. Ask the patient about physical abuse as intimate partner violence may increase during pregnancy. Ask the patient about nutrition, caffeine intake, smoking, substance use, and exercise.

Symptoms of preeclampsia include edema of hands, legs, and face; protein detected on urine dipstick; and elevated blood pressure.

Symptoms of preterm labor include uterine contractions, vaginal bleeding, and fluid leaking from the vagina.

Objective Information

Equipment Needed

Tape measure, a scale, a urine dipstick, and a fetal Doppler.

Assessment Techniques

Inspection, palpation, auscultation.

Physical Examination

The woman lies down on an examination table so that her abdomen can be examined. The healthcare provider palpates the woman's abdomen to determine the fundal height and the position and heartbeat of the fetus. Fundal height is checked by measuring from the pubic bone to the top of the uterus. Extremities are evaluated for the presence of edema.

Expected Findings

Blood pressure and fetal heart rate should be evaluated at every visit. Blood pressure should be documented at every visit. The blood pressure should not rise more than 30 points systolic or 15 points diastolic over baseline during pregnancy. The fetal heartbeat should be detected by 10-12 weeks using a fetal Doppler. The presence of a heartbeat can be detected earlier via ultrasound, approximately at the end of the first month. A normal fetal heart rate is 120-160 beats per minute.

The woman should be weighed at every visit. The total weight gain should be 20-30 lb.

The initial visit includes a complete physical examination, plus a pelvic examination.

Return visits include a blood pressure check and an abdominal examination. The abdominal examination includes checking fundal height by measuring the distance from the top of the pubic bone to the top of the uterus in centimeters (cm). After 20 weeks gestation, the fundal height in centimeters should be equivalent to the gestational age. For example, a woman who is 30 weeks pregnant should have a fundal height of 30 cm. The height is checked periodically to follow fetal growth. Before 20 weeks the growth of the uterus is evaluated in relation to landmarks in the abdomen, such as the umbilicus or the pubic bone.

After 28 weeks, it is possible to feel the fetus and determine its position in the abdomen.

Abnormal Findings

If the blood pressure becomes elevated, proteinuria or edema develop, then preeclampsia should be suspected.

Cultural Considerations

Every culture has its own traditions regarding pregnancy and childbirth. The healthcare provider is encouraged to become knowledgeable regarding the specific culture of the patient.

CASE STUDY

Lisa is a 25-year-old primigravida. She is 36 weeks pregnant. Her pregnancy has been uncomplicated. Today she denies any problems or pain. She states that her baby is moving as usual. Her blood pressure is 110/70 mm Hg and pulse is 72. She weighs 130 lb today which is a gain of 2 lb since her last visit.

Abdominal examination reveals a fundal height of 36 cm. The fetal heart rate is 140 beats per minute. There is no edema and her urine is negative for protein. The healthcare provider tells Lisa that the pregnancy is proceeding normally and that she is to return in 1 week.

REVIEW QUESTIONS

1. **The healthcare provider at the prenatal office is interviewing Lisa who is 36 weeks pregnant with her first baby. She denies any problems except that she has developed reddish brown lines on her abdomen. The healthcare provider suspects that the lines are:**
   A. striae.
   B. scratch marks.
   C. allergic reaction.
   D. a result of dry skin.

2. **As a part of the evaluation of the pregnant woman, the healthcare provider at the prenatal office should:**
   A. evaluate the patient's weight.
   B. evaluate the blood pressure.
   C. evaluate the temperature.
   D. A and B.

3. **Chloasma refers to:**
   A. the dark line that may appear from the pubic area to the umbilicus during pregnancy.
   B. the fluid that is expressed from the breasts during breastfeeding.
   C. a reddish color on the forehead and cheeks of a pregnant woman.
   D. vaginal discharge.

4. Signs of preeclampsia include:

    A. elevated blood pressure.

    B. protein in the urine.

    C. edema.

    D. all of the above.

5. The second trimester of pregnancy is:

    A. when the pregnancy test becomes positive.

    B. from conception to Week 12.

    C. from Weeks 13 to 27.

    D. from Weeks 28 to 40.

6. The hormones released by the placenta during pregnancy are:

    A. estrogen, progesterone, human placental lactogen (hPL), and human chorionic gonadotropin (hCG).

    B. cortisol, progesterone, follicle-stimulating hormone, and rennin.

    C. testosterone, luteinizing hormone, growth hormone, and aldosterone.

    D. thyroid-stimulating hormone, estradiol, prolactin, and calcitonin.

7. A pregnancy test will detect an increased level of:

    A. estrogen.

    B. progesterone.

    C. human chorionic gonadotropin (hCG).

    D. human placental lactogen (hPL).

8. Signs of preterm labor include:

    A. nausea, vomiting, and increased frequency of urination.

    B. contractions, vaginal bleeding or spotting, and leaking of fluid from the vagina.

    C. lordosis, shortness of breath, and constipation.

    D. myalgia, leg cramps, and fever.

9. A normal fetal heart rate is:

    A. 60-100 beats per minute.

    B. 100-120 beats per minute.

    C. 120-160 beats per minute.

    D. 160-200 beats per minute.

10. A fetal heart rate can first be detected by fetal Doppler at:

    A. 4-6 weeks.

    B. 6-8 weeks.

    C. 10-12 weeks.

    D. 14-16 weeks.

ANSWERS

1. A. Striae are reddish brown lines initially.

2. D. The healthcare provider should check the patient's weight and blood pressure at each office visit.

3. C. Chloasma is a reddish color on the forehead and cheeks of a pregnant woman.

4. D. Signs of preeclampsia include elevated blood pressure, proteinuria, and edema.

5. C. The first trimester lasts from Weeks 1 to 12, the second trimester from Weeks 13 to 27, and the third trimester last from Weeks 28 to 40.

6. A. Estrogen, progesterone, human placental lactogen (hPL), and human chorionic gonadotropin (hCG) are released by the placenta during pregnancy.

7. C. The hCG is the hormone detected in a pregnancy test.

8. B. Contractions, vaginal bleeding or spotting, and leaking of fluid from the vagina are all signs of preterm labor.

9. C. A normal fetal heart rate is 120-160 beats per minute.

10. C. Fetal heartbeat may be detected at 4-6 weeks by ultrasound and at 10-12 weeks by fetal Doppler.

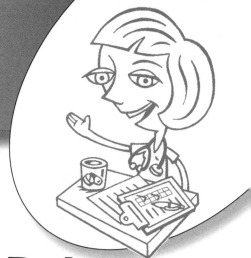

chapter 15

Assessment of Pain

LEARNING OBJECTIVES

After reviewing this chapter, the learner will be able to:

1. Identify common theories of pain.
2. Discuss the appropriate information to gather during an interview.
3. Demonstrate appropriate physical assessment techniques.
4. List normal physical assessment findings.
5. Describe abnormal physical assessment findings.
6. Discuss the age-related differences related to pain.

Review of Anatomy and Physiology

Pain receptors are located throughout the periphery. Stimulation of these pain receptors causes an (afferent) impulse to travel along the nerve fibers toward the central nervous system. There are also pain receptors on the walls of blood vessels, the pleural membranes, the peritoneal surface, and the dura mater. The body responds to an unpleasant stimulus with inflammation. The inflammatory process results in release of certain chemicals (cytokines and neuropeptides) as white blood cells, platelets, and immune cells respond to the area. The nerve fibers release substance P that enhances the transmission of the unpleasant sensation and leads to local vasodilation, increased blood flow to the area, swelling, and the release of additional chemicals (bradykinin, serotonin, and histamine).

The experience of acute pain results in a physiologic stress response that stimulates or triggers the sympathetic nervous system. This activation of the sympathetic nervous system may result in increased heart rate, respiratory rate and blood pressure, sweating, a slowed gastric emptying, elevation in blood sugar levels, pupil dilation, insomnia, anxiety, and diminished cognitive function.

Types of Pain

Chronic Pain

Chronic pain is less likely to result in changes in blood pressure, pulse rate, or respiratory rate. Patients with chronic pain are more likely to experience fatigue (which may result in irritability), insomnia, need to rest, depression, feelings of hopelessness, or social withdrawal.

Somatic Pain

Somatic pain results from messages being sent from soft tissues via nerves fibers (nociceptors) in the skin and deeper tissues. Injury or inflammation of musculoskeletal (muscle, bone, tendon, ligament, etc) will result in somatic pain. The pain is easily located and typically resolves after the injury heals. There is no actual injury to the central or peripheral nervous system. Somatic pain often responds well to conservative treatment such as ice, and over the counter antiinflammatory medications or analgesics. In some instances, the pain may become chronic.

Visceral Pain

Visceral pain originates in the internal organs. Pain receptors send the pain signal along nerve fibers (nociceptors) to the central nervous system. Compression of the organs, inflammation surrounding organs, or stretching of organs can result in pain. There is no actual injury to the central or peripheral nervous system. Visceral pain is more difficult to locate and may radiate to other areas of the body. Visceral pain is often treated with opioid medications, such as codeine (a weak opioid) or morphine (a strong opioid).

Neuropathic Pain

Neuropathic pain is caused by irritation or injury to nerve tissue. The pain can be described as sharp, burning, stinging, or pins and needles. This pain can be fairly common in conjunction with certain physiologic disorders that affect the nerves, such as diabetes. Direct damage to the nerves, as in spinal cord injuries, can lead to neuropathic pain. Localized swelling near a nerve (causing compression of the nerve) will result in neuropathic pain, as in sciatica. A variety of medications may be used for neuropathic pain. Nonsteroidal antiinflammatory medications can be helpful if swelling is involved. Antidepressant medications and anticonvulsant medications can help to alter the way in which the brain interprets the pain signal being sent.

Psychogenic Pain

Psychogenic pain is due to psychologic reasons. Although not due to physical cause, the pain is real. This pain can be more difficult to treat than pain due to a physical cause, such as inflammation. Treatments other than traditional pain medications, such as transcutaneous electrical nerve stimulation (TENS) can be utilized to manage pain. Patients with anxiety or depression may experience psychogenic pain. Complementary measures for pain control, such as distraction, can be helpful in managing psychogenic pain.

Idiopathic Pain

Idiopathic pain is a term used to classify pain when no physical or psychologic reason can be identified. The pain is real to the patient even though the cause cannot be identified. The pain can be intensified by psychologic distress. Idiopathic pain can be difficult to treat.

Acute pain is resolved relatively rapidly, within minutes, hours, days, or weeks, depending on cause. Chronic pain may result from nociceptive pain (somatic or visceral), neuropathic pain, psychogenic pain, or idiopathic pain. Chronic pain persists beyond the typical time allotted for acute pain, 3-6 months or longer. This pain may be either constant or recurrent.

The Sensation of Pain

Pain is best described as an unpleasant sensation and is primarily a subjective experience. Objective evaluation through use of standard assessment tools is necessary to properly manage a patient's pain. There are a variety of methods to objectively assess pain, including scales and physical findings. Reassessment of pain should occur following administration of an analgesic or other pain-relieving intervention. This reevaluation can help to determine the effect of the medication or intervention on the patient's pain.

Acute pain is typically of short duration, lasting for hours, days, or weeks. It is often due to a temporary condition, such as inflammation, postoperative healing, tissue trauma or damage, or other short-lived disease process. Chronic pain syndromes persist for months or years. It is commonly due to a chronic or long-standing condition, such as cancer, rheumatoid arthritis, neurologic pathology, or other long-term sequela of disease. Patients with chronic pain are often managed in a different manner than those with acute pain and may develop a tolerance to their medication, resulting in needing a higher dose or change in medication to adequately relieve their ongoing pain.

Healthcare providers need both adequate understanding of pain and preparation in pain assessment. The provider's personal experiences with pain, personal beliefs, and attitudes on pain may influence their approach to assess and manage pain.

It is important to differentiate patients who are in pain from patients who are drug seeking (those without pain who are looking for opioid medications). It is equally important to remember that patients with a history of drug use or abuse will also experience pain at times, and need to have adequate pain control options available.

Pain Theory

Gate Control Theory

Gate control theory was initially proposed in 1965. Both painful and nonpainful sensations cause transmission of the sensation along nerve fibers (see Figure 15-1). Different types of nerve fibers transmit painful and nonpainful stimulation to a relay point before sending the message to the brain. If there are more nonpainful stimuli reaching the relay point, there is no transmission of the painful sensation beyond the relay point. Then the gate is considered closed. Rubbing or holding your foot after stubbing your toe can decrease the perception of the painful stimuli as there is a greater amount of nonpainful stimuli reaching the brain. If there are a greater number of painful stimuli, then the sensation is passed through the relay point to the brain. Then the gate is considered open.

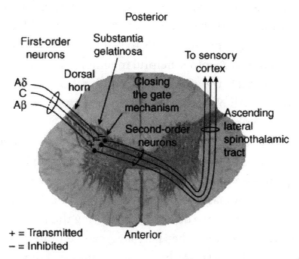

FIGURE 15-1 • Gate control theory.
(Reproduced with permission from Prentice WE, Quillen WS Underwood F: *Therapeutic Modalities in Rehabilitation*, 4th edition. New York, NY: McGraw-Hill; 2011. Figure 4-8.)

Specificity Theory

The experience of pain is processed by the brain. The pain is viewed as its own sensation which travels along nociceptors (specialized sensory receptors on peripheral nerves) in response to injury or damage.

Pattern Theory

Peripheral sensory receptors signal either nonpainful (touch, warmth, etc) or painful experiences based on the difference in patterns (timing, frequency, etc) of the signals traveling along the nerves.

Onion Theory

Multiple layers exist in this theory. At the center is the insult or injury causing the pain. The perception of pain comes next followed by suffering. Pain behavior is the next layer. There is an outer covering of interaction with the environment.

Subjective Information

Pain is a subjective experience. Ask the patient if they have any pain. Use the mnemonic OLDCARTS to remember what to ask. If pain is present, ask about the onset, location, duration, any causative or alleviating factors, radiation to other areas, the timing, and the severity of the pain. PQRST can also be used to help recall the information that needs to be elicited from the patient in pain as discussed in Chapter 1. Another helpful mnemonic is COLDSPA. Ask about the character of the pain, the onset, location, duration, severity, pattern, and any associated factors. All of these mnemonics prompt similar information and can help you to remember what to ask the patient.

A frequently used method of evaluating pain over time is to ask the patient to rate their pain on a scale of 0-10 with 0 representing no pain and 10 representing severe pain. Use of this simple evaluation can let the healthcare provider see if the pain is increasing or decreasing over time. Use of a visual analog pain scale for patients who have difficulty expressing their pain, such as a young child or patients who speak another language, can be quite helpful. The scales may show a series of faces (from happy to crying) or color variations (with green or blue representing comfort and transitioning to red which typically represents pain).

Review of Systems (ROS)

Ask the patient about the pain. Also try to determine if the pain is having an effect on other systems or daily activities. Sleep, food intake, activity level, family responsibilities, ability to concentrate, mood, and sexual function can all be altered by pain.

Risk Factors Related to Pain

Physiologic disorders may increase the risk for pain. Patients with musculoskeletal injury or disease are likely to have somatic pain. Disorders that cause inflammation or alteration in blood flow to internal organs increase the likelihood of visceral pain. Diabetes increases the risk for neuropathic pain. Mental health disorders, such as depression or anxiety, increase the chances that the patient will experience psychogenic pain. Patients with chronic pain syndromes have a greater chance of developing depression.

Risk Evaluation

Ask the patient about the presence of pain and its characteristics. Screen the patient with chronic pain for depression.

Self-Care Behaviors

Patients should be taught to notice the triggers to pain and to act appropriately. For example, if the patient has an aura (a premonition) before a migraine headache, the patient should initiate appropriate treatment as recommended by their healthcare provider. Medication prescribed for pain should be taken when the pain begins. The patient should not wait until the pain is severe to take prescribed medication, because it will take longer to experience relief of the pain. The patient who is experiencing pain should be taught to tell the healthcare provider immediately when the pain begins and to report new onset of pain or a change in the pain which could signal a problem.

Objective Information

Patients often exhibit physiologic signs that they are experiencing pain. The patient may look uncomfortable or distressed or their vital signs may be different from their normal readings. In patients with chronic pain, vital signs are not a good indicator of pain.

Equipment Needed

Blood pressure cuff, watch, visual analog pain scale.

Assessment Techniques

Inspection and Palpation

First, ask the patient if they are experiencing any pain. Find out where the pain is located and when it began. Ask the patient to describe the pain (sharp, dull, throbbing, burning, gnawing, etc). Allow the patient to select the appropriate word to describe the sensation; do not lead their answer by offering to describe what you think they are feeling. Ask what makes the pain better or worse.

Inspect the area of pain if possible. Gently palpate the area, taking care not to cause any unnecessary increase in the level of pain.

Physical Examination

Vital signs: Check the patient's vital signs. During pain or distress, the blood pressure, pulse rate, and respiratory rate may all increase.

Inspection and Palpation

Look at the patient's facial expressions for signs of discomfort. Examine the area where the patient complains of pain. Assess the skin for discoloration and even pigmentation. Look for lesions, swelling, ecchymosis, or breaks in the skin. For musculoskeletal disorders, evaluate the patient's ability to move normally. Is any movement restricted due to discomfort? Inspect the joints and muscles for pain with movement (see Chapter 10). Inspect the area for any signs of inflammation (redness or swelling) or ecchymosis (black and blue discoloration of the skin).

Patients with visceral pain may have difficulty localizing the pain, or the pain may appear to move. The patient with appendicitis can initially have pain in the periumbilical area rather than in the right lower quadrant of the abdomen, where the appendix is located.

Some patients with neurogenic pain due to neurologic damage may be unaware that they have altered sensory perception in the affected areas. Check for sensation. Use of a monofilament to check for touch perception is an easy way to assess the area (see Figure 15-2). Touch the monofilament to the skin and apply gentle pressure until the filament begins to bend. The patient should be aware of the touch with this light pressure. Testing perception of warmth and cold is also necessary for patients with neurogenic pain. You can use test

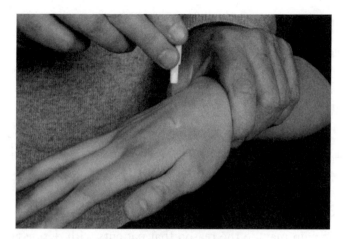

FIGURE 15-2 • Monofilament to check for touch perception.
(Reproduced with permission from Dutton M: *Dutton's Orthopaedic Examination, Evaluation, and Intervention*, 3rd edition. New York, NY: McGraw-Hill; 2012. Figure 18-68.)

tubes filled with hot and cold water to check the patient's ability to determine temperature differences. If the test tube with the hot water is too hot for you to hold, it is too hot to rest against the patient's skin. Vibratory sensation may also be compromised. Use a tuning fork with a low pitch (128 Hz) to check for vibration perception. Strike the tuning fork against the heel of your hand while holding it by the handle. Contact with the vibrating tines of the tuning fork will impede the vibration. Place the handle of the tuning fork over the most peripheral bony prominence, such as the distal interphalangeal joint. The patient should be able to sense the vibration (see Chapter 11).

Expected Findings

Somatic Pain

It is often related to disease or injury affecting the skin and deeper tissues. Performance of simple tasks (walking, completion of activities of daily living [ADLs]) may be impaired. Associated swelling and warmth may occur with musculoskeletal injury.

Visceral Pain

It is often difficult to localize and may radiate to other areas of the body. Pain may be described as general, such as diffuse abdominal pain, rather than in a specific location.

Neuropathic Pain

It often involves the periphery, such as the feet. Normal sensation may be impaired due to the pain. Walking may be affected due to this altered sensation.

Idiopathic Pain

Idiopathic pain, while real to the patient, does not have a noted physiologic cause and is often more difficult to manage. Patients can easily become frustrated when testing is unable to find a cause for their pain.

Psychogenic Pain

Psychogenic pain may be the reason that patients with depression or anxiety first seek treatment.

Abnormal Findings

Assess the patient's overall comfort level. Their facial expression may indicate discomfort or pain. Difficulty concentrating or irritability may be due to the level of pain the patient is experiencing. Some patients may avoid eye contact when they are uncomfortable. The patient may be sitting or lying in a way that diminishes the pain. The healthcare provider may note that the patient appears to be protecting (or guarding) a painful area. If physical abnormal signs are not present, it is still important to believe the patient's symptoms of pain.

Age-Related Changes

Pediatric

Small children often have difficulty expressing or describing pain. Using physiologic cues of distress can be helpful in assessing the patient for pain. Children may become irritable or attempt to self-soothe (rocking, curling up, being uncharacteristically quiet, wanting to be held, or left alone) or exhibit other behavior that is not typical. Use of visual analog pain scales can aid in evaluation of the pain and effectiveness of treatment.

Geriatric

Some older patients view pain as a normal occurrence of aging and may not think to mention their discomfort. Others may have had earlier experiences with pain that impact their current experiences with pain. Somatic pain is fairly common as people age. Visceral pain signals may be blunted. An older patient may have significant disease (eg, a ruptured appendix) with only mild to moderate pain.

Cultural Considerations

People from different cultures react to pain in different ways. Some cultures are very verbal about the pain that is experienced. In some instances, making noise (moaning, talking, etc) can be viewed as beneficial to aid in pain relief. Other cultures remain very stoic, despite significant pain levels. A variety of factors contribute to how a patient experiences, reacts to, and attempts to control pain. Family lessons, earlier experiences with pain and its management, and personal meaning of pain all impact the patient's perception of and reaction to pain. It is important to take cues from the patient and their experience and preferences in dealing with pain and not use your own perception or experience with pain to judge what the patient is feeling or how they should be responding.

CASE STUDY

Ms A is a 21-year-old college student who was walking down a flight of stairs earlier today and twisted her right ankle. She is now complaining of pain in her right ankle when she tries to put pressure on it. There is positive swelling on the lateral aspect of the ankle. Ms A is concerned that she will not be able to continue her classes at the local university. Ms A states she is willing to follow medical advice so she can return to classes as soon as possible.

REVIEW QUESTIONS

1. **Ms A's pain would be:**
   A. somatic.
   B. visceral.
   C. neuropathic.
   D. psychogenic.

2. **Ms A's pain would likely be treated with:**
   A. topical application of ice.
   B. an opioid medication.
   C. transcutaneous electrical nerve stimulation (TENS).
   D. warm soaks.

3. Patients with chronic pain are likely to exhibit which of the following?
   A. Increased heart rate, respiratory rate, and blood pressure.
   B. Insomnia, fatigue, depression, feelings of hopelessness.
   C. Sweating, elevation in blood sugar levels, dilated pupils.
   D. Diminished cognitive function, slowed gastric emptying, anxiety.

4. Where is substance P released from?
   A. Blood vessels
   B. Spinal cord
   C. Nerve fibers
   D. Pleural membranes

5. The type of pain when no physical or psychologic reason can be recognized is called:
   A. somatic pain.
   B. psychologic pain.
   C. false pain.
   D. idiopathic pain.

6. Ms A is from a culture that does not express pain by crying or moaning. Instead Ms A believes that she should endure pain silently. What should the healthcare provider do to help Ms A?
   A. Not offer pain relief until Ms A asks for something to relieve the pain.
   B. Allow Ms A to suffer silently because of her cultural beliefs.
   C. Explain the pain severity scale to Ms A.
   D. Avoid Ms A because she is not complaining of pain.

7. Why should the healthcare provider take Ms A's vital signs?
   A. To document the vital signs in the medical record.
   B. The vital signs may change for the patient in pain.
   C. All patients in pain have an increase in the pulse rate.
   D. It is an expected order from a physician.

8. What is the difference in pain sensation in the young adult as compared with the older adult?
   A. The older adult has decreased pain sensation levels.
   B. The younger adult complains about pain more frequently.
   C. The older adult is stoic when discussing pain levels.
   D. The younger adult has difficulty understanding pain scales.

9. **What should the healthcare provider do if physical signs of pain are not assessed?**
   A. Ignore the patient's requests for pain medication.
   B. Return to reassess the patient in 2 hours.
   C. Assess the patient for illicit drug abuse.
   D. Believe the patient and offer pain relief methods.

10. **Which of the following pain theories advise rubbing the affected area to relieve pain?**
    A. Specificity theory
    B. Pattern theory
    C. Gate control theory
    D. Onion theory

ANSWERS

1. A. Ms A's pain would be somatic because the pain is originating from the swelling in the soft tissue of the ankle via nerve fibers (nociceptors) within the tissues.

2. A. Somatic pain is best treated with topical application of ice. An ice pack should be applied to the area with a thin towel or material between the skin and the ice to avoid damage of the skin by the extreme cold. Ice is applied for the first 48 hours for 20 minutes on and 20 minutes off.

3. B. Patients with chronic pain are more likely to experience fatigue (which may result in irritability), insomnia, need to rest, depression, feelings of hopelessness, or social withdrawal.

4. C. The nerve fibers release substance P that enhances the transmission of the unpleasant sensation and leads to local vasodilation, increased blood flow to the area, swelling, and the release of additional chemicals (bradykinin, serotonin, and histamine).

5. D. Idiopathic pain is a term used to classify pain when no physical or psychologic reason can be identified. The pain is real to the patient even though the cause cannot be identified.

6. C. Explain the severity scale to Ms A and advise her to tell the healthcare provider her pain level. Assess Ms A's pain level often and offer pain relief methods as needed. After Ms A receives pain medication or other relief methods return, to assess if the pain level has decreased.

7. B. The vital signs in a patient may change if the patient is experiencing an increase in pain.

8. A. Pain is blunted in the older adult and they may not complain about severe pain with significant disease entities.

9. D. If physical abnormal signs are not present, it is still important to believe the patient's symptoms of pain.

10. C. Gate control theory—rubbing the area of pain will close the gate and decrease the perception of the painful stimuli, because there is a greater amount of non-painful stimuli reaching the brain.

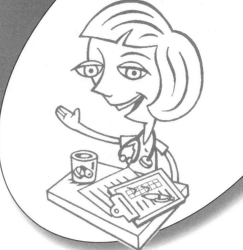

chapter 16

The Head to Toe Comprehensive Assessment

After reviewing this chapter, the learner will be able to:

1. Discuss the appropriate subjective information to gather during an interview.

2. Demonstrate a comprehensive physical assessment.

3. List normal physical assessment findings.

4. Describe abnormal physical assessment findings.

5. Discuss the important age-related differences.

KEYWORDS

Bronchophony
Ectomorphic
Endomorphic
Extraocular movements (EOMs)
Gallop

Guarding
Mesomorphic
Murmur
Point of maximal impulse (PMI)
Rebound

Introduction

Now that you have reviewed each body system, the time has come to put them all together in an organized manner. Collection of subjective data occurs first as this helps you to focus your attention on a specific area or identify risk factors pertinent to the patient. You want to develop a systematic approach so that you are able to include all the necessary assessment techniques while limiting any unnecessary discomfort or positional changes for the patient.

Review of Anatomy and Physiology

Consider the underlying anatomic structures when performing your physical examination. Knowledge of anatomic landmarks assists you in performing the necessary skills.

Subjective Information

Begin by introducing yourself and determine how the patient prefers to be addressed. It is better to ask the patient about their preference, rather than assuming that you know how to address the patient.

Interview

Ask the patient why they are seeking care today. If there is a complaint, ask specific questions to find out more about their symptoms. Determine the onset, duration, location, contributing and alleviating factors, presence of any radiation of pain, the timing and setting in which the symptom occurs. Ask the patient what they think may have caused their symptoms. This can help to identify the patient's frame of reference for their current condition.

Determine significant risks for the patient. Risks may include actual or potential disease states or lifestyle factors that increase health risk. Ask the patient about their history. This includes medical, social, and family history. Medical history includes any chronic or significant acute illnesses. Ask about any earlier surgical procedures. Ask if the patient takes any medications and if they know the dosage. Ask about allergies and what reaction occurs. Determine if the patient has received recommended vaccinations. Social history includes daily living and lifestyle choices. Ask about occupation and whether any recommended safety equipment is actually used. Ask about substance use which includes alcohol, smoking, or drug use. Ask about illicit drug use and inappropriate use of prescription medications. Patients may take prescription medications (such as pain medications) that were intended for someone else without realizing the risks involved. Ask about recreational hobbies and determine if recommended safety equipment is used. Ask about living arrangements and if the patient has a support system. Family history should include the members of the family and their ages, any illnesses experienced, and the cause of death and age for those who are deceased. A family history should include three generations (the patient's generation and two others). Inquire about any siblings, the parents, and grandparents (if known) or the patient's children (if appropriate).

Review of Systems (ROS)

A ROS is completed to determine if there are other significant problems besides what the patient is seeking care for currently. Begin by asking about general state of well-being (fatigue, unexplained weight changes, etc) and move onto specific body systems. Whenever the patient gives a positive response, you will need to investigate the symptom further (onset, duration, location, etc).

Head and neck–Ask about headaches, lightheadedness, swollen glands, neck pain (and whether it occurs with or without movement), or any injuries to the area.

Eye, ear, nose, and throat–Ask about visual changes (blurring, floaters, changes in peripheral vision), discomfort, itching or discharge, changes in hearing (loss, tinnitus) or balance, nasal congestion, sinus pressure, nasal discharge, sore throat, voice changes, or any trauma to these areas.

Cardiovascular–Ask about any chest discomfort or palpitations, varicose veins, claudication (cramping pain in the calf that occurs with exercise and resolves with rest), cold hands, and/or feet.

Respiratory–Ask about shortness of breath (and whether it occurs at rest or only with exertion), cough (with or without sputum production), wheezing, dyspnea on exertion.

Gastrointestinal–Ask about indigestion, nausea, vomiting, diarrhea, constipation, any changes in bowel patterns (such as change in bowel habits, or color or consistency of stool), pain, or bloating.

Genitourinary–Ask about any discomfort with urination, frequency, urgency, changes in urinary patterns, flank pain, urethral discharge, or blood in the urine.

Male–Ask about urethral discharge, lesions in the genital area, scrotal discomfort or edema, determine if the patient performs testicular self-examination (and if not, ask if they know how to perform the examination), ask about safe sex practices and sexual preference (men, women, or both), and the number of partners (an increase in sexual activity puts the patient at an increased risk of sexually transmitted diseases).

Female–Ask about urethral or vaginal discharge, menstrual cycle changes, breast discomfort, determine if the patient performs breast self-examination (and if not, ask if they know how to perform the examination), ask about safe sex practices and sexual preference (men, women, or both) and the number of sexual partners.

Musculoskeletal–Ask about any joint pains, muscle aches, limitation of movements, gait disturbances, or injuries to the joints.

Skin–Ask about any lesions, changes in skin color, or texture or changes in moles. Any of these may be a sign of skin cancer, which occurs more commonly on sun-exposed skin. Benign skin lesions may also occur. Ask about wounds that heal slowly, as these may also signify skin cancer or a systemic illness such as diabetes.

Hematologic and lymphatic–Ask about unusual bleeding or bruising, or swollen glands.

Objective Information

Equipment Needed

Gloves, ophthalmoscope, otoscope, stethoscope, tongue depressor, cotton swab, tuning fork, thermometer, blood pressure cuff, watch, soft centimeter ruler.

Assessment Techniques

Inspection, auscultation, palpation, and percussion.

Physical Examination

Complete a general survey to inspect the patient's overall appearance. Look at posture, skin color, respiratory effort, and facial expression. Does the patient appear to be in any distress? Does the patient appear to be their stated age? Assess their body habitus. Do they appear to be well nourished (mesomorphic), underweight (ectomorphic), or overweight (endomorphic)?

Heent–Inspect the patient's head. Are there any lesions, inflammation, areas of hair loss, or signs of injury? Look at the scalp beneath the patient's hair. Are there any nits or lice present? Palpate the skull for areas of tenderness or malformation.

Inspect the face for symmetry. Note any loss of muscle mass in the temporal areas. Check the eyes for symmetry or any signs of inflammation. Use an external light (penlight or ophthalmoscope) to check the pupil reaction to light. Determine symmetry of visual fields. Assess the extraocular movements (EOMs) of the eyes. Ask the patient to raise their eyebrows, close their eyes, and frown. Ask the patient to keep their eyes tightly shut while you gently attempt to open them. Inspect the conjunctiva for any irritation or drainage by gently displacing the eyelid. Inspect the inner structure of the eye using the ophthalmoscope, beginning with the red reflex. Locate the optic disc and the vessels, following them to all four quadrants. Inspect the ears for location, symmetry. Palpate the external ear for tenderness or lesions. Gently displace the external ear by pulling up and back in adults or down and back in infants and toddlers to straighten the ear canal to allow for better visualization of the canal and tympanic membrane. Use the otoscope to inspect the ear canal and tympanic membrane. Inspect the nose for appearance and discharge. The septum should be midline. The nasal mucosa should be pink and moist. Ask the patient to smile and then puff out their checks checking for symmetry. Inspect the mouth and throat. The oral mucosa should be pink and moist. Inspect the teeth for any signs of caries or missing teeth. Inspect the soft and hard palate. Note any lesions or malformations. Inspect the posterior pharynx and tonsilar areas. The tonsils are located between the anterior and posterior pillars in the lateral oropharynx. Inspect the uvula. It should be midline and remain midline (should not deviate to either side) when the patient says "aahhhh" which will raise the soft palate.

Inspect the neck for any abnormalities, swelling, or lesions. Palpate the carotid pulse, first on one side, then the other. Gently palpate the lymph nodes in the neck noting the consistency, any tenderness, enlargement, and mobility. Ask the patient to swallow while inspecting the anterior neck to help locate the thyroid gland. Gently palpate the thyroid, noting consistency, symmetry, or any nodules. Ask the patient to flex and extend the neck, tilt the head toward one shoulder and then the other, and turn the head side to side to assess range of motion (ROM). Ask the patient to turn their head to the side while you place your hand against their cheek to provide resistance. Ask the patient to shrug their shoulders.

Listen over the carotid area to determine whether there is a bruit noted. There is lack of consistency in recommendations to use either the bell or the diaphragm of the stethoscope for optimal identification of a carotid bruit. Since sources are contradictory, best practice would be to use both (first one, then the other), making sure to avoid unnecessary pressure on the artery.

Chest–Inspect the chest for any signs of injury and symmetry of respirations. Gently palpate the anterior chest noting any tenderness, particularly at the costosternal junction. Palpate the posterior chest for tenderness, including the spinous processes. Place your hands along the chest wall in the lower thoracic area, first posteriorly and then anteriorly. Have the patient take a deep breath and note the movement of the chest wall (watch to see how far your hands move apart with inhalation and toward each other with exhalation) with both inspiration and exhalation. Palpate the chest with the medial (pinky) side of your closed fist as the patient says "ninety- nine." Mild vibration is considered normal. Locate the point of maximal impulse (PMI). The PMI is typically found in the apical area. In adults, this should be located in the fifth intercostal space (ICS) in the midclavicular line. Note any unusual vibration (thrill) as you gently palpate at the second ICS on the left and right borders of the sternum, and the third, fourth, and fifth ICSs at the left sternal border and the fifth ICS in the midclavicular line. Percuss the chest, both anteriorly and posteriorly. You should hear resonance on percussion over the lung fields. Use a systematic pattern as you move along the chest wall, alternating between the right and left sides to assess for symmetrical findings. Auscultate the anterior chest with the bell of the stethoscope, following the same pattern that you used for percussion, alternately listening to the right and left sides of the chest. Make sure you check the right middle lobe area that can only be assessed anteriorly or laterally. Auscultate the anterior chest with the diaphragm of the stethoscope. Auscultate the posterior chest diaphragm of the stethoscope. If you note any abnormal breath sounds, assess transmitted breath sounds. Ask the patient to say "ninety-nine" as you listen to the chest in the concerning area. The words should sound muffled. If the words are clear (bronchophony), there is an increased likelihood of consolidation in the area. Also ask the patient to say "E" as you listen to the chest in the concerning area. In an area of consolidation, the spoken "E" will sound like "ay" (egophony). Listen to the heart sounds through the anterior chest. Use the bell and then the diaphragm of the stethoscope to listen to cardiac sounds on the anterior chest at the second ICS at the right and left sternal border, the third, fourth, and fifth ICSs and in the fifth ICS at the midclavicular line. Note which sounds are present and the regularity of the rhythm. Normal heart sounds have an S1 and S2 component. Extra sounds should be noted as to the anatomic location and timing within the cardiac cycle, whether systolic or diastolic.

Abdomen–Assess the uncovered abdomen for contour, vascular pattern, or any signs of peristaltic movement or vascular pulsations. Auscultate over all four quadrants to assess both bowel sounds. Note the frequency and pitch of the bowel sounds. If the bowel sounds are infrequent, leave the stethoscope in one place for up to 5 minutes before you determine that the bowel sounds are absent. Assess the vascular sounds over the midline upper abdomen (aorta), on the right and left side near the costal margins (renal arteries), and the lower abdomen about midway between the umbilicus and groin (iliac arteries). The vascular sounds should have a similar sound to a distant heartbeat. A swishing sound is a bruit. It is important to auscultate the abdomen before palpating or percussing, as you want to be sure that the bowel sounds you hear are naturally occurring and not the result of your manipulation. Percuss over the abdomen, noting areas of dullness. Dullness is a normal finding over solid organs, such as the liver or spleen. Gently palpate the abdomen for any tenderness. Perform a more thorough assessment by deep palpation of the abdomen. Note any areas of tenderness, masses, guarding (protecting the area of discomfort), or rebound (an increase in pain when releasing the pressure of palpation).

Percuss over the costovertebral angle (the angle created by the 12th rib meeting the vertebrae). There should be no tenderness here. Gently palpate the suprapubic area for tenderness or presence of a full bladder. Palpate deeply over the upper abdomen, within the costal angle (the angle created by the lower ribcage, as the ribs join the sternum). Examine the urethral meatus for any signs of discharge. Ask the patient for a urine sample, noting the color, clarity, and any odor of the urine.

Musculoskeletal–Each joint should be assessed in a systematic fashion, working from head to toe and comparing right to left for symmetry. Inspect the temporomandibular joint (TMJ) area for swelling or signs of injury. The area can be gently palpated while the patient opens and closes their mouth.

There should be no clicking or pain upon opening or closing of the mouth on examination. Inspect the neck for muscle tone, swelling, or signs of injury. Palpate the spinous processes in the posterior neck for muscle tone, pain, or swelling. Ask the patient to actively demonstrate ROM of the neck by tilting the head back to look overhead, lowering their chin toward their chest, turning the head to the right and the left, tilting their ear toward each shoulder and rotating the head.

Inspect the shoulder for muscle tone, swelling, or signs of injury. Palpate the landmarks of the shoulder (head of the humerus, acromium process, acromioclavicular joint, subacromial bursa) for muscle tone, swelling, or discomfort. There should be no tenderness or swelling noted on palpation. Ask the patient to actively demonstrate ROM of the shoulders by holding their arms straight out in front with arms parallel to the floor and the palms down, then rotate to have the palms up, raise the arms overhead, rotate the arms back to form a full circle, raise the arms to the sides and then overhead, cross the arms to touch the opposite hips, and touch the upper back (near the scapula) of the opposite side of the body. Inspect for muscle tone, swelling, or signs of injury to the elbow. Palpate the elbow (olecranon process, medial and lateral epicondyles, medial and lateral tendon grooves) for muscle tone, discomfort, or swelling. Ask the patient to flex and then extend the elbow. Ask the patient to hold their lower arm horizontal to the floor with the palms facing up, and then rotate the hand so the palms face the floor. Inspect the wrist and hand for muscle tone, inflammation, or signs of injury. Patients with long-standing carpal tunnel syndrome will have a loss of muscle tone in the thenar eminence (the area between the base of the thumb and the midline anterior wrist). Palpate the wrist, palm, and fingers for muscle tone, tenderness, or swelling. Ask the patient to flex, extend, abduct, adduct, and rotate the wrist. Ask the patient to make a fist and then open the hand, extending the fingers. Ask the patient to spread the fingers, bring them together, touch each finger to the thumb on the same hand, and oppose the thumb by touching it to the fifth finger.

Inspect the back for muscle tone, swelling, signs of injury, and for symmetry of scapular and hip height. Note the normal curvature of the spine in the cervical, thoracic, lumbar, and sacral areas. Palpate the spinous processes for tenderness or swelling. Ask the patient to stand up with feet together and bend forward with the hands together, touching the toes. Note the appearance of the spine. There should be no lateral deviation of the spine and the scapula and hips should be at the same height.

Inspect the hips for swelling or signs of injury. Palpate the bony landmarks and the bursae of the hip joint. Assess active ROM of the joints with the patient standing (if balance and stability are not a concern) or lying on an examination table or bed (may be active or passive). The hip should allow the following motions: abduction (move away from midline), adduction (move toward midline), flexion (bending), extension (straightening), medial rotation (turning toward midline), lateral rotation (turning away from midline). The movements should be fluid and without discomfort.

Inspect the knees for swelling or signs of injury. Palpate the bony landmarks of the knee, checking for swelling or tenderness. Assess ROM by asking the patient to extend and straighten the lower leg.

Inspect the ankles and feet for swelling or signs of injury. Palpate the bony landmarks for swelling, tenderness, or abnormal motion. Assess ROM of the ankle for flexion, extension, rotation, inversion, and eversion. Ask the patient to flex, extend, and spread the toes noting any lesions in between the toes or discolorations.

Abnormal Findings

Additional assessment of certain areas may be indicated if abnormalities are identified. Each chapter describes both the expected and unexpected findings for each body system.

Head–Note any asymmetry of the head or evidence of trauma. Note area of alopecia (loss of hair) or thinning of the eyebrows.

Neck–Neck pain at rest or on movement would be abnormal and warrants further examination. Determine if the pain is present only with active motion or also with passive movement. Do the muscles in the posterior neck and shoulder area feel tight? A sprain or muscle spasm will produce pain, but is not life-threatening. Nuchal rigidity refers to difficulty with neck motion due to the spasm and rigidity of the neck muscles. Pain on movement is a different symptom. Check for meningeal irritation by having the patient lie in a supine position on the examination table or bed and flex their neck (chin moving toward chest). A positive sign is increased pain with movement and flexion of knees and hips due to discomfort. Kernig sign also indicates meningeal irritation and is elicited by having the supine patient flex the hips and knees to a 90 degree angle. Pain is produced when the healthcare provider attempts to extend the lower leg. Neck pain due to meningeal irritation is typically accompanied by photophobia (sensitivity to light) and headache.

A bruit (signifying turbulence of blood flow) may be heard over the carotid arteries.

Eyes, Ears, Nose, and Throat (EENT)–Eye drainage may be the result of infection (such as conjunctivitis) or irritation of the eye. Visual field defects may be found when there is damage to the retina or brain (result of a cerebrovascular accident [CVA] or trauma). Visual loss may be due to trauma, damage to the retina or brain (inability to perceive images), glaucoma (as a result of increased intraocular pressure—there is a loss of peripheral vision), and macular degeneration (there is a loss of central vision). Hearing loss is more common as people age, with the loss of higher tones more prevalent. Hearing loss is more pronounced in those who have had sustained exposure to loud noises. Pain is a symptom and the location, onset, duration, and aggravating and alleviating factors need to be established. Drainage from the ear may be due to an infection within the ear canal or perforation of the tympanic membrane. Pharyngitis (inflammation of the throat) is commonly due to a viral infection, but may also occur with bacterial infections (such as strep), postnasal drip, or inhaled irritants. Swollen glands typically occur as a result of localized infection. These glands will be tender, mobile, and enlarged. Enlarged glands that are fixed, hard, or nontender are more concerning for serious illness. The thyroid may have palpable nodules or appear larger than anticipated.

Cardiac–Pulse rate may be higher than expected, which is referred to as tachycardia, or slower than expected, which is referred to as bradycardia. The heart rhythm can be regular or irregular. If it is regular, it is important to note whether it is regularly irregular (every third beat is skipped) or irregularly irregular. Extra heart sounds may be present such as an S3, S4, gallop, murmur, or rub. An S3 sound occurs in early diastole (filling) and may be due to fluid overload or left ventricular systolic dysfunction. An S4 sound is late in diastole and may be found in patients with uncontrolled hypertension. A gallop is the addition of S3 and/or S4 sounds. A murmur is produced when there is turbulence of blood flow. Note the location and timing of the murmur. A rub is produced by friction. You can differentiate a pulmonary friction rub from a cardiac friction rub by asking the patient to hold their breath. If the rub continues, it is cardiac.

Respiratory–Asymmetry of movement occurs when the chest is not expanding equally. This may be due to injury (trauma to the area or fractured ribs) or pain (such as with pleurisy). Look for the use of accessory muscles (abdominal breathing in an adult, intercostal or supraclavicular retractions). Inspect for cyanosis and determine if it is central or peripheral. Palpate for increased fremitus due to consolidation (as in pneumonia), tenderness (possibly due to localized trauma or inflammation). Listen for abnormal breath sounds (due to the presence of fluid, wheeze, inequality of air exchange, stridor, rub) or transmitted breath sounds (bronchophony, egophony, whispered pectoriloquy).

Abdomen–Listen for abnormal timing of bowel sounds (hypoactive or hyperactive) or the presence of a bruit. Palpate for areas of tenderness, rebound, or guarding, which may be due to inflammation or infection within the abdomen.

Musculoskeletal–Assess for limited ROM or point tenderness on palpation of the joints.

Age-Related Changes

Pediatric

A systematic approach to interviewing and physical examination is recommended regardless of the age of the patient. Minor adjustments to your approach are appropriate to better accommodate the developmental needs of the younger patients.

Interaction with children makes knowledge of normal growth and development essential. Physical examinations can cause fear in children as they may not know what to expect, or may perceive the equipment as unfamiliar and frightening. Including the child's caregiver can ease the uncertainty of younger children. Explaining the examination as you go about it can also help to ease concerns of both the child and the caregiver. Also, allowing children to touch the equipment can make the equipment less frightening to them.

Geriatric

Older patients are typically more familiar with the information gathering (interview) and physical examination techniques. You may need to position yourself facing the patient when asking questions or speak more slowly to enhance comprehension of those who have difficulty hearing. Some older patients may need more time to process information to answer the questions. Limitation in vision or hearing is more common as people age. Difficulty with movements due to joint pains or arthritis is also more common in geriatric patients.

Cultural Considerations

Being sensitive to the individual patient's culture and personal needs is necessary when examining them. Protecting the patient's privacy as well as attending to any specific cultural matters is important to their sense of comfort during the examination.

Family involvement varies from one culture to another. Some cultures are very paternalistic with the eldest male having great influence on decisions that are made. Some cultures honor the older members of the family, showing them great respect. Other cultures avoid conflict and respect authority figures and may be uncomfortable in questioning or disagreeing with a healthcare provider's recommendations. Some patients do not want to be asked what course of treatment should be undertaken; they prefer to be told what should be done.

Disease may be viewed based on belief in a scientific effect, as the result of pathology or infection. Some cultures believe that an imbalance in energy may be the cause of their current symptoms. A belief in the effect of hot and cold forces explains the use of some home remedies. Some patients rely on prayer or other spiritual rituals when faced with illness, and may view disease as a punishment for some wrongdoing.

CASE STUDY

Andy is a 27-year-old professional who is returning to college to obtain a graduate degree and needs to have a complete physical check-up for student health clearance as part of the process.

REVIEW QUESTIONS

1. **When beginning the encounter with a new patient, it is best to:**
   A. introduce yourself and ask the patient how they would like to be addressed.
   B. start with the physical examination and then interview the patient.
   C. always address the patient by their first name to show that you are being friendly.
   D. instruct the patient on the importance of smoking cessation.

2. **If the patient is seeking care for a specific complaint (such as abdominal pain), the healthcare provider should elicit:**

    A. what the patient believes is the cause of the complaint.

    B. whether anything has made the symptom better or worse.

    C. details about the complaint, such as the onset, duration, location, presence of radiation, timing, and setting and severity of the symptom.

    D. all of the above.

3. **When asking the patient about their history, you include the:**

    A. medical and surgical history.

    B. social history.

    C. family history.

    D. all of the above.

4. **A Review of Systems (ROS) is conducted to:**

    A. organize the order of the physical examination.

    B. determine if there are any other significant problems that need to be addressed.

    C. identify risk for disease based on the patient's family history.

    D. identify substance abuse.

5. **When you first encounter the patient, the healthcare provider should complete a general survey to evaluate the patient's overall appearance. This should include looking at their body habitus, posture:**

    A. skin color, respiratory effort, and facial expression.

    B. skin temperature and texture and hair texture.

    C. spinal alignment, range of motion (ROM) of extremities, and presence of cyanosis.

    D. pupillary reaction to light, appearance of the tympanic membrane, and abdominal girth.

6. **An endomorphic body type is:**

    A. underweight.

    B. normal weight.

    C. overweight.

7. **When interviewing an older patient, the healthcare provider should:**

    A. allow the patient to touch or play with the equipment before the examination.

    B. face the patient when asking questions.

    C. gather information from the chart since that patient probably does not remember the answers to the questions.

    D. turn on the radio for background noise to maintain patient privacy when asking questions.

8. **Which of the following would be normal findings on the physical examination?**
Select all that apply.

   A. regular heart rate and rhythm, 2+ peripheral pulses bilaterally equal, no pulse deficit.

   B. bowel sounds in all four quadrants, abdomen soft and nontender to palpation.

   C. chest expansion symmetrical, respirations even and unlabored, lungs clear to auscultation.

   D. tenderness to palpation of right costosternal border.

9. **Costovertebral tenderness is properly assessed by:**

   A. quickly releasing your hand when palpating the abdomen to check for the presence of pain.

   B. placing the hands on the lower thoracic and note the movement when the patient breathes.

   C. percussing over the area where the 12th rib meets the vertebral column.

   D. gently palpating the lymph nodes in the neck.

10. **Which of the following would be considered an abnormal finding?**

    A. A bruit present when listening to the carotid artery.

    B. A heart rate of 112 in an adult patient.

    C. Rhonchi noted in the right middle lobe.

    D. A systolic murmur noted on the left sternal border best heard at the fourth intercostal space (ICS)

    E. All of the above.

ANSWERS

1. A. Always introduce yourself to the patient before beginning an examination. The healthcare provider should call the patient by their preferred name whenever possible.
2. D. You should find out as much detail as you can about the current symptom(s).
3. D. Medical, surgical, social, and family history are all part of the patient's history.
4. B. A Review of Systems (ROS) is completed to determine if there are any other significant problems that need to be addressed.
5. A. Body habitus, posture, skin color, respiratory effort, and facial expression are all included in the general survey.
6. C. An endomorphic body type is overweight.
7. B. Face the patient when asking questions to assist those who may have difficulty hearing.

8. A, B, and C. A regular heart rate and rhythm, 2+ peripheral pulses bilaterally equal, no pulse deficit; bowel sounds in all four quadrants, abdomen soft and nontender to palpation; and chest expansion symmetrical, respirations even and unlabored, lungs clear to auscultation are all normal findings on physical examination.
9. C. Costovertebral angle tenderness is assessed by percussing over the area where the 12th rib meets the vertebral column.
10. E. All of these findings are considered abnormal.

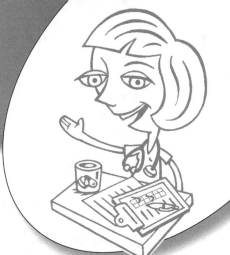

chapter **17**

Comprehensive Review Questions

1. The healthcare provider is preparing to interview a new patient. At what distance should the healthcare provider be to facilitate comfort for the patient?

   A. 1-2 feet
   B. 3-4 feet
   C. 6-8 feet
   D. 4-6 feet

2. Which of the following is an example of false reassurance?

   A. uh huh, go on.
   B. Describe your pain.
   C. Don't worry it will be ok.
   D. How old are you?

3. The question "You do not smoke cigarettes do you?" is an example of which of the following?

   A. Misleading question
   B. Open-ended question
   C. Closed-ended question
   D. Conversational question

4. The patient's sexual preference(s) should be documented in which of the following areas?

   A. Family history
   B. Social history
   C. Past history
   D. Self-care behaviors

5. A patient returns to the clinic for the healthcare provider to check a wound that occurred 3 days ago. The type of assessment needed is:

   A. comprehensive assessment.
   B. emergency assessment.
   C. focused assessment.
   D. follow-up assessment.

6. At what time of the day is the temperature of a patient higher than average?

   A. Late morning
   B. Early afternoon
   C. Early morning
   D. Late afternoon

7. The healthcare provider should assess the pulse of a patient for which of the following? *Select all that apply.*

   A. Warmth
   B. Rate
   C. Rhythm
   D. Amplitude
   E. Elasticity

8. Where is the popliteal pulse found in the adult patient?

   A. In the groove between the medial malleolus and the Achilles tendon.
   B. Dorsum of the foot, below proximal to and parallel to the great toe.
   C. Deep in the soft area of the posterior knee.
   D. Under the inguinal ligament in the groin area.

9. An adult who has a respiratory rate of less than 12 breaths a minute would be documented by the healthcare provider as?

   A. Eupnea
   B. Tachypnea
   C. Bradypnea
   D. Dyspnea

10. **Which of the following is an important procedure to follow when using electronic equipment to take a patient's blood pressure?**

    A. Ensure that the blood pressure cuff is two times the width of the patient's arm.
    B. Always use electronic equipment, if the patient's pulse is irregular.
    C. The equipment needs to be calibrated according to the manufacturer's instructions.
    D. Abnormal readings should be rechecked in 10 minutes using electronic equipment.

11. **The layer of the skin that provides insulation for heat regulation is which of the following?**

    A. Epidermis
    B. Dermis
    C. Subcutaneous
    D. Appendages

12. **Palpation of the skin reveals which of the following properties of the skin? *Select all that apply.***

    A. Edema
    B. Turgor
    C. Texture
    D. Moisture
    E. Temperature

13. **An angle of greater than 180 degrees of a patient's nail would reveal an abnormality called?**

    A. Paronychia
    B. Clubbing
    C. Koilonychia
    D. Onycholysis

14. **Acne that develops in puberty is associated with:**

    A. protein deficiency.
    B. poor hygiene.
    C. increase in sebum production.
    D. decrease in androgens.

15. **An irregular-shaped scar formed after injury to the skin that develops from excessive collagen production is called:**

    A. a keloid.
    B. a chloasma.
    C. a melasma.
    D. a cyst.

16. The patient flexes the neck with the chin toward the chest and reveals which of the following?

    A. Third intercostal space
    B. First thoracic vertebrae
    C. 12th free floating rib
    D. Seventh cervical vertebrae

17. The healthcare provider is conducting an interview of a patient who is short of breath. It is essential for the healthcare provider to:

    A. provide a laundry list of answers for all questions.
    B. ask open-ended questions at this time.
    C. stabilize the patient before asking for a complete health history.
    D. ask questions that require an explanation.

18. A patient states that he has smoked two packs of cigarettes a day for 20 years. This would be documented as:

    A. 20 pack-years.
    B. 30 pack-years.
    C. 40 pack-years.
    D. 10 pack-years.

19. The healthcare provider percusses the thorax over the right lung and discovers a dull area instead of resonance. This could indicate which of the following?

    A. Consolidation
    B. Rhonchi
    C. Air in the bronchi
    D. Obstruction in the trachea

20. The outer-most layer of the heart is the:

    A. myocardium.
    B. pericardium.
    C. endocardium.
    D. epicardium.

21. The sound generated when the tricuspid valve and the mitral valve close is called?

    A. S3
    B. S2
    C. S1
    D. S4

22. The patient wakes up suddenly after being asleep for 2-4 hours and feels short-ness of breath and needs to sit or stand to relieve the shortness of breath. This is documented as:

    A. dyspnea on exertion.
    B. orthopnea at rest.
    C. bradypnea with exercise.
    D. paroxysmal nocturnal dyspnea

23. The process of atheromas (fatty deposits) in the intimal lining of arteries *begins* with:

    A. accumulation of calcium.
    B. thrombi formation.
    C. endothelial injury.
    D. necrosis of cardiac tissue.

24. The patient complaints of dizziness upon arising from a supine position to a sitting or standing position. This is called:

    A. toxic hypertension.
    B. orthostatic hypotension.
    C. lightheadedness.
    D. pulsus paradoxus.

25. The healthcare provider is assessing the anterior chest of a 25-year-old patient at the second intercostal space to the right of the sternum. This area is termed the:

    A. aortic area.
    B. pulmonic area.
    C. tricuspid area.
    D. mitral area.

26. Which of the following organs of the abdomen are considered solid viscera?

    A. Pancreas, kidneys, bladder
    B. Stomach, colon, small intestines
    C. Liver, spleen, pancreas
    D. Ovaries, uterus, gallbladder

27. What is the function of the stomach?

    A. Convert glucose to glycogen.
    B. Filter metabolic waste products.
    C. Absorb water and form stool.
    D. Store and digest food.

28. **Which is the best method to assess a patient's food intake?**

    A. Ask the patient for a list of all foods eaten in the past 24 hours.
    B. Ask the patient if he/she eats fast/junk food on a daily basis.
    C. Ask the patient to describe carbohydrates, proteins, and fats.
    D. Ask the patient if he/she has had symptoms of constipation recently.

29. **Mr Smith is an 85-year-old patient who lives alone on a limited income. The healthcare provider is performing a nutritional assessment. Which of the following questions would assess Mr Smith's nutritional status?**

    A. Do you like to eat meat, potatoes, and vegetables?
    B. Do you shop for your own food and prepare it yourself?
    C. Do you smoke cigarettes every day?
    D. How many glasses of alcohol do you consume daily?

30. **What can the healthcare provider do to relax the patient's abdominal muscles during an abdominal assessment?**

    A. Ask the patient to breath in and out through the mouth.
    B. Perform the examination from the right side of the bed.
    C. Perform deep palpation after light palpation.
    D. Place a pillow under the patient's knees.

31. **The healthcare provider performs indirect percussion on the posterior thorax at the level of the 12th rib to assess which of the following organ(s)?**

    A. Kidneys
    B. Liver
    C. Spleen
    D. Large intestine

32. **An observation of a scaphoid abdomen is assessed by the healthcare provider and can be found in which of the following conditions?**

    A. Ascites
    B. Malnutrition
    C. Organ enlargement
    D. Intraabdominal bleeding

33. **The healthcare provider places a hand at a 90 degree angle on the left lower quadrant of the abdomen and presses deeply and quickly releases the hand. The patient states that the abdominal pain increased on the right side of the abdomen. This sign is called:**

    A. Cullen sign
    B. Rebound tenderness
    C. Murphy sign
    D. Rovsing sign

34. The patient states that he has lactose intolerance, and therefore he has intolerance to which of the following foods?

    A. Meats
    B. Dairy
    C. Fruits
    D. Spicy

35. Which of the following is the definition of a ligament?

    A. Joins bones to other bones at the joint.
    B. Place where a bone meets cartilage at a joint.
    C. Where bones are connected to muscles.
    D. Type of bone cell that breaks down bone.

36. The healthcare provider asks the patient to move the right arm away from the midline of the body. This movement is called?

    A. Flexion
    B. Inversion
    C. Adduction
    D. Abduction

37. During a musculoskeletal assessment interview, it is important for the healthcare provider to ask questions about which of the following?

    A. Intake of protein and fats.
    B. Activities of daily living.
    C. Problems with vision.
    D. Shortness of breath on exertion.

38. The healthcare provider is interviewing a 55-year-old postmenopausal woman. Which of the following would reduce her risk of osteoporosis?

    A. Having a bone density examination.
    B. Taking a daily multivitamin.
    C. Eating 3 oz of protein daily.
    D. Weight-bearing exercises.

39. The patient complains of his right shoe wearing quicker than his left shoe. What could this indicate?

    A. Foot fracture
    B. Uneven gait
    C. Bunions
    D. Sprained ankle

40. Which of the following joint abnormalities is a decreased or complete immobility of a joint?

   A. Subluxation
   B. Dislocation
   C. Ankylosis
   D. Contracture

41. Which of the following patients has the highest risk of fractures?

   A. A 41-year-old Hispanic woman.
   B. A 75-year-old African American man.
   C. A 55-year-old Caucasian woman.
   D. A 50-year-old African woman.

42. The organ that stores and allows spermatozoa to fully mature is which of the following?

   A. Epididymis
   B. Testes
   C. Corpus cavernosa
   D. Prostate

43. A patient complains of pain on urination. The healthcare provider would document this as:

   A. pyuria.
   B. aciduria.
   C. nocturia.
   D. dysuria.

44. The patient complains of discharge in the urine. Which of the following should the healthcare provider ask about the discharge? *Select all that apply.*

   A. Color
   B. Amount
   C. Odor
   D. Consistency
   E. Discomfort

45. One of the risk factors that put the patient at a risk of contracting a sexually transmitted disease is which of the following?

   A. Use of a condom
   B. Multiple partners
   C. Monogamous relationship
   D. Use of a dental dam

46. **The healthcare provider is percussing over a full bladder. The sound expected when percussing over a full bladder is:**

    A. resonance.
    B. tympany.
    C. dullness.
    D. flatness.

47. **If lymph nodes are palpable, which of the following characteristics would be considered benign?** *Select all that apply.*

    A. Tender
    B. Mobile
    C. Rubbery
    D. Hard
    E. Small

48. **What occurs in Tanner Stage 2 of puberty in a male?**

    A. Pubic hair becomes darker and coarser.
    B. The penis increases in width as well as length.
    C. Enlargement of the testicles and scrotum.
    D. The penis becomes longer but not wider.

49. **It is documented in the medical record as "primigravida" for Ms Smith. The healthcare provider understands that this refers to which of the following?**

    A. Ms Smith has had three miscarriages.
    B. She is pregnant for the first time.
    C. The patient has had two past pregnancies.
    D. Her pap smear evaluation is up to date.

50. **The term used to define areas of increased pigmentation on the forehead, cheeks, and nose during pregnancy is called?**

    A. Chloasma
    B. Stretch marks
    C. Striae
    D. Linea nigra

51. **During the third trimester, it is common for the woman to develop which of the following due to the altered center of gravity?**

    A. Kyphosis
    B. Scoliosis
    C. Barrel chest
    D. Lordosis

52. Ms Jones comes to the clinic complaining of "missed menses." The *initial* question the healthcare provider should ask Ms Jones is:

   A. the date of her last menstrual period (LMP).
   B. if she uses condoms during intercourse.
   C. number of earlier pregnancies.
   D. if she desires an abortion.

53. The healthcare provider suspects a 35-week pregnant female to have preeclampsia. Which of the following are signs of preeclampsia? *Select all that apply.*

   A. Blood in urine and stool.
   B. Vaginal bleeding.
   C. Elevated blood pressure.
   D. Protein detected in urine.
   E. Edema of hands, legs, and feet.

54. Which of the following are signs of sympathetic nervous system activation? *Select all that apply.*

   A. Increased blood pressure.
   B. Slowed gastric emptying.
   C. Decreased heart rate.
   D. Low blood sugar levels.
   E. Pupils dilate.

55. Which of the following can be a cause of visceral pain?

   A. Compression or inflammation of an organ.
   B. Injury to the peripheral nervous system.
   C. Irritation or injury to nerve tissue.
   D. No physical or psychologic reason.

56. Mr M is a 35-year-old male who used illicit drugs in the past. He comes to the clinic complaining of severe abdominal pain. Which of the following would be the best action by the healthcare provider?

   A. Suspect he is drug seeking.
   B. Assess his level of pain.
   C. Avoid the use of all opioids.
   D. Reassess him in 1 hour.

57. The healthcare provider is using the mnemonic "OLDCARTS" to assess a patient's pain. The *first* question to ask the patient would be?

   A. Is the pain stabbing or dull?
   B. Can you point to the pain?
   C. What relieves the pain?
   D. When did the pain start?

58. The *initial* area of pain associated with appendicitis is commonly located in which part of the abdomen?

    A. Suprapubic
    B. Epigastric
    C. Periumbilical
    D. Right lower quadrant

59. A 5-year-old female patient is crying and has both arms placed across the abdomen. The healthcare provider can evaluate her pain level by using which of the following?

    A. Initial pain scale
    B. Brief pain inventory
    C. Visual pain scale
    D. Auditory pain scale

60. A healthcare provider would use the monofilament tool to assess which of the following?

    A. Sensory perception
    B. Reflexes
    C. Motor function
    D. Clonus

61. Which cerebral lobe is associated with emotions, personal behaviors, and impulse control?

    A. Frontal lobe
    B. Parietal lobe
    C. Occipital lobe
    D. Temporal lobe

62. The 12 cranial nerves have fibers that originate in the:

    A. cerebellum.
    B. cerebrum.
    C. brainstem.
    D. spinal cord.

63. The daughter of a patient reports that "Mom continuously eats spoiled food." Which cranial nerve should the healthcare provider assess for?

    A. Cranial nerve I, olfactory
    B. Cranial nerve II, optic
    C. Cranial nerve III, oculomotor
    D. Cranial nerve V, trigeminal

64. A patient complains of coughing after eating and noticed a loss of taste. Which cranial nerve should the healthcare provider assess?

    A. Cranial nerve IX, glossopharyngeal
    B. Cranial nerve VIII, vestibulocochlear
    C. Cranial nerve XI, spinal accessory
    D. Cranial nerve XII, hypoglossal

65. What are the components of the physical examination? *Select all that apply.*

    A. Inspection
    B. Palpation
    C. Percussion
    D. Auscultation
    E. Observation

66. Clubbing is associated with which of the following?

    A. Lung cancer or cystic fibrosis
    B. Chronic bronchitis
    C. Asthma
    D. Emphysema

67. Tactile fremitus, a palpable breath sound, is _____ by trapped air or pleural fluid and _____ by consolidation.

    A. decreased, increased
    B. increased, decreased
    C. decreased, decreased
    D. increased, increased

68. Which type of adventitious lung sound has a crackling sound heard mid to late inspiration?

    A. Rhonchi
    B. Wheezes
    C. Rub
    D. Fine crackles

69. What is the least expensive way to assess if a patient is in respiratory distress?

    A. Arterial blood gas.
    B. Inspection on physical examination.
    C. CT scan of the lung.
    D. Chest X-ray.

70. **As a healthcare provider, you function as:**
    A. an advocate for the patient.
    B. a healthcare proxy for the patient.
    C. the power of attorney for the patient.
    D. a legal representative for the patient for healthcare decisions.

71. **Nonverbal communication skills include:**
    A. awareness of the patient's personal space preferences.
    B. respecting differing preferences for touch and eye contact, based on cultural awareness.
    C. awareness of one's own body position when talking with the patient.
    D. all of the above.

72. **The healthcare provider observes that the patient has recently been crying. Which of the following is an appropriate response to the patient at this time?**
    A. "You look upset, would you like to talk about it?"
    B. "Don't worry; I'm sure that everything will be fine."
    C. "Let me tell you about what happened to me earlier today."
    D. Avoid the patient as crying makes you uncomfortable.

73. **The nursing process offers a framework to identify needs, create a plan of care, and determine the effectiveness of the interventions. Which of the following stages of the nursing process involves the assessment of which interventions were successful and which ones were not?**
    A. Assessment
    B. Diagnosis
    C. Planning
    D. Evaluation

74. **During a review of systems (ROS), patients are asked about the presence of specific symptoms. A helpful mnemonic to elicit further information about symptoms that are present is PQRST. This stands for:**
    A. Place or position, quality and quantity, radiation, severity and setting, and timing and treatments.
    B. Provider of healthcare, quality of care received, referrals made to specialists, system involved, and treatments recommended.
    C. Parent's health history, quotient of health, rendered treatment, specialists actually seen, tolerance of treatments rendered.
    D. Presence, quantity, referral of symptom to other location, setting in which the symptom occurs, trust in care given.

75. The patient provides a list of the current medications, vitamins, and herbal supplements taken at home. This is included in:

    A. subjective data.
    B. objective data.
    C. care plan.
    D. assessment.

76. Extraocular movements (upper and lower lateral and medial movement of the eyes) are controlled by cranial nerve(s):

    A. I
    B. III, IV, and VI
    C. V and VII
    D. IX and X

77. Checking a bicep reflex assesses neuromuscular function at the level of:

    A. C5-C6
    B. C7-C8
    C. L2-L4
    D. S1

78. A diminished deep tendon reflex would be appropriately described as:

    A. 0
    B. 1+
    C. 2+
    D. 3+

79. The ability to eat is necessary for survival. In assessing an infant, the healthcare provider is aware that the following cranial nerves are involved in sucking and swallowing:

    A. I.
    B. III, IV, and VI.
    C. V, VII, IX, X, and XII.
    D. all of the above.

80. The healthcare provider is assessing cortical sensation in a patient and asks the patient to close their eyes and traces the letter A on the patient's palm. It is correctly identified. This is documented as which of the following is intact?

    A. Stereognosis
    B. Two-point discrimination
    C. Graphesthesia
    D. Point location

81. **When performing a neurologic assessment, the healthcare provider should:**
    A. position yourself on the right side of the patient.
    B. use a cephalocaudal approach.
    C. start with the patient in a supine position.
    D. speak loudly and slowly while facing the patient.

82. **The submental node is correctly palpated:**
    A. in the midline, just below the bony area of the chin.
    B. behind the external ear, slightly above the mastoid process.
    C. behind the sternocleidomastoid muscle.
    D. anterior to the tragus.

83. **Tinnitus may develop:**
    A. following damage to the acoustic nerve.
    B. as a result of exposure to loud noises.
    C. due to head trauma.
    D. all of the above.

84. **Visual loss associated with glaucoma typically:**
    A. results in loss of central vision.
    B. begins with loss of peripheral vision.
    C. is age related and results in difficulty focusing on near objects.
    D. results in difficulty in differentiating colors.

85. **A patient that is stuporous is considered to be:**
    A. not arousable, no response to painful stimuli.
    B. minimal spontaneous activity, withdrawal response to painful stimuli.
    C. sleepy, slowed responses.
    D. drowsy, mumbling responses.

86. **With patients that have no response to verbal stimuli, select an appropriate action to attempt to elicit a response?** *Select all that apply*
    A. Pinching the skin between the thumb and index finger.
    B. Pinching the lower portion of the nail.
    C. Yell in the patient's ear till a response is elicited.
    D. Stop further assessment as the patient is purposely ignoring the provider as she/he is desperate to get some rest.

87. When assessing abnormalities within a patient's speech, which key term(s), refer to uncontrollable repetition of words? *Select all that apply.*

    A. Echolalia
    B. Perseveration
    C. Selective mutism
    D. Clang associations

88. The term "Loose association" refers to:

    A. a rapid flow of speech jumping from topic to topic that is unrelated.
    B. a disordered thought process, where a series of ideas have a lack of logical connection.
    C. a disorganized thought process that lacks meaning and coherence.
    D. an irrational, unshakable belief that something is true when it is not.

89. The term "hallucination" refers to:

    A. a sensation of something that appears to be real but is not, and may include tactile, auditory, olfactory sensations.
    B. inappropriate perception of a stimulus that is real, but is not properly interpreted.
    C. a perception of being personally threatened or impending harm.
    D. none of the above.

90. Long-term use of combination (estrogen-progestin) hormonal therapy has been linked to: *Select all that apply.*

    A. increased risk of heart attack.
    B. increased risk of stroke.
    C. increase risk of blood clot formation.
    D. decreased risk of breast cancer.

91. Menorrhagia is a medical term that describes:

    A. an abnormally heavy flow.
    B. an irregular pattern.
    C. an abnormally heavy flow that is irregular.
    D. absence of menstrual bleeding.

92. The patient comes in with a complaint of a vaginal discharge that is gray with a fishy odor. Which of the following would the healthcare provider suspect?

    A. *Candida* infection
    B. Gonorrhea
    C. Trichomoniasis
    D. Bacterial vaginosis

93. Gravida is the term that refers to:

    A. the number of times a woman has been pregnant regardless of the outcome.

    B. the number of deliveries.

    C. the number of abortions or miscarriages.

    D. the number of live children.

94. Human papillomavirus (HPV) has been linked to which type of cancer(s)?

    A. Cervical cancer

    B. Vulvar and vaginal cancer

    C. Penile and anal

    D. Oropharyngeal cancers

    E. All of the above

95. The healthcare provider is assessing a 25-year-old female with a chief complaint of abdominal pain. Which of the following questions would assess pain level?

    A. Does the pain radiate to your lower back?

    B. On a scale of 1-10, can you rate the pain?

    C. Do you feel nauseous when you have the pain?

    D. What relieves the abdominal pain?

96. The healthcare provider assesses a patient and needs to document the following vital signs: Blood pressure 120/80 mm Hg, pulse 80, respirations 20, temperature 98.6 orally. Which of the following is the *best* documentation?

    A. Vital signs are normal.

    B. WNL (within normal limits) vital signs.

    C. Obtained vital signs.

    D. Document actual values.

97. Which of the following are methods of validating data? *Select all that apply.*

    A. Ask the patient's family if the information is true.

    B. Repeat the assessment.

    C. Clarifying the information with the patient.

    D. Verify with a more experienced healthcare provider.

    E. Look for clarification of information on the Internet.

98. If the healthcare provider wants to change an entry in a medical record, which of the following would be the correct method to change the record?

    A. "White out" the entry and rewrite the correct entry.

    B. Cross out the entry several times and write over the top of the original entry.

    C. Cross the incorrect entry with one line and write "mistake in entry."

    D. Blacken the incorrect wording with a marker and continue writing.

99. **Which method of palpation would be used to assess a patient with pendulous breasts?** *Select all that apply.*

    A. Light palpation
    B. Deep palpation
    C. Bimanual palpation
    D. Moderate palpation

100. **Which of the following is considered objective data?** *Select all that apply.*

    A. Complains of abdominal pain.
    B. Pain upon palpation of abdomen.
    C. Feels nauseous after eating fish.
    D. Positive rebound tenderness.
    E. Vomited after eating dinner.

ANSWERS

1. B. Most patients would prefer the healthcare provider to be about 3-4 feet away.

2. C. Don't worry it will be ok is an example of false reassurance. A is an example of facilitation, B is an open-ended statement seeking information, and D is a closed-ended question.

3. A. asking the patient "You do not smoke cigarettes do you?" could embarrass the patient if he/she is smoking cigarettes and is misleading the patient to state "No."

4. B. The patient's sexual preference(s) should be documented in the social history.

5. D. Assessment after a health problem has been identified with review of present concerns and identification of any new concerns. It establishes a diagnosis in need of follow-up care.

6. D. The patient's temperature in the early morning is lower than average and is higher than average in the late afternoon or evening.

7. B, C, D, E. The healthcare provider assesses the pulse for rate, rhythm, amplitude, and elasticity of the pulse.

8. C. Deep in the soft area of the posterior knee. A is the posterior tibial pulse. B is the dorsalis pedis pulse. D is the femoral pulse.

9. C. Breathing less frequently than normal (<12 breaths per minute in the adult) is bradypnea. A is within normal range of breathing, B is breathing more frequently than normal (>20 breaths per minute in the adult), and D is difficulty with breathing.

10. C. The equipment needs to be calibrated according to the manufacturer's instructions. A, B, and D are false.

11. C. The subcutaneous layer consists of connective tissue and adipose tissue that supports the outer layers of the skin. This layer provides insulation for heat regulation. The epidermis layer protects the skin and along with elastin and collagen strengthens the skin. The dermis layer nourishes the epidermis by papillae from the

dermis that project into the epidermal region. Hair and nails are considered append-ages of the skin, and serves to protect the body and filter dust and other debris.

12. A, B, C, D, and E. All of the answers are correct and are revealed when the health-care provider palpates the skin.

13. B. Clubbing is the proximal edge of the nail elevated to greater than 180 degrees associated with long-standing oxygen deprivation to the periphery.

14. C. In puberty, increase in sebaceous gland activity with resultant increase in sebum production, increase in androgens, and bacteria on the skin produce acne.

15. A. Keloids are irregular shaped-scars formed after injury to the skin, which develop from excessive collagen production. It is a condition that is probably hereditary due to the fact that it is common in certain families. The scar is not cancerous but can cause cosmetic problems for the patient.

16. D. The most prominent vertebral process is the seventh cervical vertebra or C7. This is easily located as it is the most prominent vertebral process noted when the patient flexes the neck (chin toward chest).

17. C. Ask only short-answer questions and stabilize the patient before asking a com-plete health history or open-ended questions. It would not be advisable to provide a laundry list to all questions at this time, because it would prolong the interview before the patient received interventions to relieve the shortness of breath.

18. C. Multiply the packs of cigarettes smoked per day times the number of years the patient smoked. (Packs per day) × (years of smoking) = pack-years.

19. A. Percussion over an area of consolidation will cause a dull sound.

20. B. The outer-most layer of the heart is the pericardium, which consists of an outer fibrous layer and a thin inner layer.

21. C. The sound generated when the tricuspid valve and the mitral valve close is called S1.

22. D. Paroxysmal nocturnal dyspnea (PND) occurs when the client wakes up suddenly after being asleep for 2-4 hours and feels shortness of breath and needs to sit or stand to relieve the shortness of breath.

23. C. Atheromas (fatty deposits) develop in the intimal wall of the coronary arteries. This happens in a progressive fashion with the process beginning with endothelial injury and a focal deposit of cholesterol and lipids.

24. B. A complaint of dizziness upon arising from a supine position to a sitting or standing position is termed as orthostatic hypotension.

25. A. The healthcare provider should auscultate the anterior chest at the four areas where the valves of the heart radiate as follows:

   1. Aortic area: Second intercostal space to the right of the sternum.
   2. Pulmonic area: Second intercostal space to the left of the sternum.
   3. Tricuspid area: Left sternal border at the fourth or fifth intercostal space.
   4. Mitral area: Apex of the heart at the fourth or fifth intercostal space, midcla-vicular line.

26. C. The internal organs of the abdomen are called the viscera and consists of solid viscera, which maintain a characteristic shape: liver, spleen, pancreas, kidneys, ovaries, uterus, adrenal glands, and the hollow viscera, which change shape based on contents inside (such as bladder, gallbladder, stomach, small intestine, colon).

27. D. Functions to store, and digests food by the secretion of necessary enzymes and churning motions.

28. A. The best method to assess a patient's food intake is to ask for a 24-hour diet recall of a typical day.

29. B. Older adults can have difficulty going to the store and preparing meals.

30. D. Placing a pillow under the patient's knees will relax the abdominal muscles.

31. A. Kidneys—the healthcare provider performs indirect percussion posteriorly at the level of the kidneys at the costovertebral angle (CVA) at the 12th rib by placing one hand flat against the back at the level of the 12th rib and strike that hand with the medial side of the closed fist on the other hand.

32. B. A scaphoid abdomen may be seen in a patient with progressive disease or malnutrition.

33. D. The Rovsing sign or referred rebound tenderness.

34. B. Patients who cannot tolerate dairy foods are considered lactose intolerant and are possibly lacking the enzyme lactase that helps to digest dairy products.

35. A. The ligaments join bones to other bones at the joints.

36. D. Abduction is the movement of an extremity away from the midline of the body.

37. B. The interview of a patient for the musculoskeletal system focuses on activities of daily living (ADLs) and functional assessment, as well as specific questions about the bones, joints, and muscular function.

38. D. Weight-bearing exercises will help prevent osteoporosis.

39. B. Shoes that are worn unevenly could reveal an uneven gait.

40. C. Ankylosis is a decreased or complete immobility of a joint due to the fusion of the bones of the joint, commonly caused by trauma, disease, or chronic inflammation.

41. C. Hispanics and people of African descent have a higher bone density than Caucasians. Therefore, Caucasian women have a higher incidence of fractures of the spine and hip.

42. A. Within the epididymis are spermatic ducts where the spermatozoa that have been produced, can be stored, and allowed to fully mature.

43. D. Dysuria is discomfort with urination. Pyuria is pus in the urine, aciduria is abnormal amounts of acid in the urine, and nocturia is excessive urination at night.

44. A, B, C, D. The healthcare provider should ask about color, amount, odor, and consistency of the discharge. Pain is an associated question usually related to urination and not the discharge.

45. B. Multiple partners will put the patient at risk of contracting a sexually transmitted disease.

46. C. Dullness is expected over a full bladder. Resonance is heard over lung tissue, tympany is heard over the abdomen, and flatness over a bone.

47. B, C, and E. Normal lymph nodes are small (<0.5 cm), nontender, rubbery, and mobile. A hard lymph node could indicate malignancy and tenderness could indicate infection.

48. C. The second phase is when the first visible signs of puberty occur, there is enlargement of the testicles and scrotum, and pubic hair begins to develop at the base of the penis. Pubic hair becomes darker and coarser and the penis becomes longer (but not wider) during Stage 3, and during Stage 4 the penis increases in width as well as length.

49. B. A woman pregnant for the first time is referred to as a primigravida. A woman who has been pregnant more than once is referred to as a multigravida.

50. A. The face may develop areas of increased pigmentation on the forehead, cheeks, and nose. This is known as chloasma. Striae or stretch marks may develop on the abdomen and breasts. These initially appear as reddish brown lines. After the pregnancy they may change color to silvery white. It is common for the woman to develop a dark line of pigmentation from the pubic area to the upper abdomen. This line is called the linea nigra.

51. D. The increased abdominal area weight in an advanced pregnancy alters the center of gravity for the expectant mother and results in a wider stance and lordosis (increased curvature of the lumbar area of the back). Kyphosis is an exaggerated thoracic curvature of the spine, scoliosis is a lateral curvature of the spine, and barrel chest is when the transverse diameter and the anterior-posterior diameter of the chest are equal instead of 2:1.

52. A. The first question the healthcare provider should ask the patient is the date of her last menstrual period (LMP).

53. C, D, and E. Symptoms of preeclampsia include edema of hands, legs, and face; protein detected on urine dipstick; and elevated blood pressure. Symptoms of preterm labor include uterine contractions, vaginal bleeding, and fluid leaking from the vagina.

54. A, B, and E. Activation of the sympathetic nervous system results in increased heart rate, respiratory rate and blood pressure, sweating, slowed gastric emptying, elevation in blood sugar levels, pupil dilation, insomnia, anxiety, and diminished cognitive function.

55. A. Visceral pain originates in the internal organs. Pain receptors send the pain signal along the nerve fibers (nociceptors) to the central nervous system. Compression of the organs, inflammation surrounding organs, or stretching of organs can result in pain. There is no actual injury to the central or peripheral nervous system. Neuropathic pain is caused by irritation or injury to nerve tissue and idiopathic pain is a term used to classify pain when no physical or psychologic reason can be identified.

56. B. All patients should be assessed for pain level and treated accordingly. It is important for the healthcare provider to believe the patient before assuming he is drug seeking.

57. D. Using the mnemonic OLDCARTS, ask the patient in pain about the **o**nset, **l**oca-tion, **d**uration, any **c**ausative or **a**lleviating factors, **r**adiation to other areas, the **t**iming, and the **s**everity of the pain.

58. C. Patients with visceral pain may have difficulty localizing the pain, or the pain may appear to move. The patient with appendicitis can initially have pain in the periumbilical area rather than in the right lower quadrant of the abdomen, where the appendix is located.

59. C. A visual scale, for example, faces with smiles to frowns can best evaluate a child's pain level when the child is unable to state the level of pain using a 0-10 pain scale.

60. A. The monofilament is used to test sensory perception. Touch the monofilament to the skin and apply gentle pressure until the filament begins to bend. The patient should be aware of the touch with this light pressure. To assess reflexes use a reflex hammer, to assess motor function ask the patient to move the tested area through the full range of motion, and to test clonus rapidly dorsiflex the foot and look for rapid, rhythmic contractions of the leg muscle.

61. A. The frontal lobe. The parietal lobe is responsible for sensory control, visual, olfac-tory, and auditory sensation; the occipital lobe is responsible for interpreting visual data; and the temporal lobe is responsible for processing and interpreting auditory stimuli.

62. C. The 12 cranial nerves, which are peripheral nerves, have fibers that originate in the brainstem.

63. A. Cranial nerve I. Cranial nerve I assesses the olfactory nerve. Smell can alert a patient if the food has been spoiled. Cranial nerve II assesses for visual acuity, whereas cranial nerve III assesses the extraocular movement with eye opening and pupil constriction and cranial nerve V is the trigeminal nerve that tests for facial sensation.

64. A. Cranial nerve IX, glossopharyngeal affects the gag reflex and taste on the pos-terior portion of the tongue. Coughing after eating may be a sign that the patient's gag reflex is not functioning. Cranial nerve VIII, vestibulocochlear affects the ability to detect sounds. Cranial nerve XI, spinal accessory assesses lateral head move-ment and trapezius strength, and cranial nerve XII, hypoglossal affects tongue movement.

65. A, B, C, and D. Observation is part of inspection.

66. A. Clubbing is associated with diffuse fibrosis of the lung. It is frequently seen in cystic fibrosis and associated with lung cancer. It is not a sign of asthma, emphy-sema, or chronic bronchitis.

67. A. Fremitus is decreased by pleural fluid or trapped air (eg, pneumothorax/air in the pleural space), and is increased by consolidation.

68. D. Crackles or rales have a crisp crackling sound, and thus the name "crackles" which indicate fluid in the alveoli or fibrosis of the lung. Whereas Rhonchi is a coarse sound caused by turbulence of airflow around mucus in larger airways, wheezes have a whistling sound due to airflow within the narrowing of airways, and a rub has a harsh scratching sound caused by an inflamed pleural surface.

69. B. The healthcare provider can most efficiently assess, with the lowest cost, if a patient is in respiratory distress by inspection on physical examination. Signs of respiratory distress are increased respiratory rate and use of accessory muscles.

70. A. A healthcare provider is an advocate for the patient.

71. D. All of these are components of nonverbal communication.

72. A. Validate the patient's current status and offer the opportunity to talk about it. Avoid false reassurances or changing the focus to you.

73. D. Evaluation of the plan of care allows the healthcare provider to make adjustments to the plan if needed.

74. A. When the patient has a positive response when asked about the presence of a symptom, it is important to determine more information about the symptom—where, when, how much, and what type of symptom, whether it travels to another area, and which treatments have already been tried.

75. A. Information provided by the patient is subjective information.

76. B. Cranial nerves III, IV, and VI control extraocular movements. The sense of smell is related to cranial nerve I. Cranial nerves V and VII control facial sensation and movement. Cranial nerves IX and X innervate the soft palate.

77. A. Bicep and brachioradialis reflexes assess C5-C6. Patellar reflexes assess L2-L4. Achilles reflex assesses S1.

78. B. 0 describes absence of a deep tendon reflex; 1+ describes a diminished reflex; 2+ describes a normal reflex; 3+ describes an increased reflex.

79. C. Cranial nerve I is involved in the sense of smell. Cranial nerves III, IV, and VI are involved in extraocular movements. Cranial nerves V, VII, IX, X, and XII are involved in sucking and swallowing.

80. C. Stereognosis is the ability of the patient to identify common objects by touch. Two-point discrimination is tested by the ability of the patient to differentiate between one and two points of contact. Graphesthesia is the ability of the patient to identify a letter or number traced on their palm. Point location describes the ability of the patient to locate the area being touched.

81. B. A cephalocaudal approach is typically used for a neurologic assessment.

82. A. In the midline, just below the bony area of the chin.

83. D. Tinnitus may be the result of acoustic nerve damage, head trauma, or exposure to loud noises.

84. B. Visual loss associated with glaucoma typically begins with loss of peripheral vision.

85. B. Minimal spontaneous activity, withdrawal response to painful stimuli.

86. A and B are appropriate actions to attempt to elicit a response.

87. A and B. Echolalia and perseveration has uncontrollable repetition of the same words. Selective mutism occurs when a person who is capable of speech is unable to speak, and clang associations describe a connection between words or ideas based on the sound.

88. B. A flight of ideas refers to a rapid flow of speech jumping from topic to topic that appears to be unrelated. A word salad describes a thought process that is disorganized, lacking coherence and meaning, and delusions are irrational, unshakable belief that something is true when it is not.

89. A. Illusions occur when the perception of a stimulus is real but is not properly interpreted, whereas paranoia refers to the perception of being personally threatened or feeling that someone or something is "out to get" or harm you.

90. A, B, and C. Long-term use of hormonal therapy increases an individual risk for cardiovascular disease (such as heart attack and stroke), breast cancer, and blood clot formation. D is incorrect because hormonal therapy increases the risk of breast cancer, not decreases it.

91. A. Menorrhagia is an abnormally heavy menstrual flow. Metrorrhagia is the term used when menstrual cycles occur with an irregular pattern. Menometrorrhagia is the term used when there is prolonged or abnormally heavy bleeding that occurs irregularly and more frequently than normal. Amenorrhea is the absence of menstrual bleeding.

92. D. A white to gray discharge with a fishy odor is typical of bacterial vaginosis. A thick, white, curd-like discharge is typical of a *Candida* (yeast) infection. Cloudy white or yellow may indicate gonorrhea. Trichomoniasis infection typically has a frothy, yellow-green discharge with a noticeable odor.

93. A. Gravida is the number of times a woman has been pregnant; para is the term which refers to the number of deliveries. Abortus/abortion refers to spontaneous abortions or miscarriage.

94. E. There are over 150 strains of human papillomavirus (HPV), and are associated with vulvar, vaginal, penile, anal, and oropharyngeal cancers.

95. B. The pain scale is one of the best methods to determine the pain level of the patient.

96. D. The best documentation for vital signs is to document the exact values. Avoid the use of the word normal or WNL (within normal limits), and the healthcare provider does not need to state that the vital signs were performed.

97. B, C, and D. Repeating the assessment, clarifying the information with the patient, and verifying with a more experienced healthcare provider are all methods of validating data. It is not necessary to ask the family if the patient is alert and oriented to time, person, and place, and the Internet can have incorrect information.

98. C. Cross the incorrect entry with one line and write "mistake in entry." The other answers are incorrect methods of correcting a medical record.

99. C and D. Bimanual palpation would be used, in addition to moderate palpation.

100. B and D. Pain on palpation of abdomen and positive rebound tenderness are objective data, and A, C, and E are subjective data.

Index

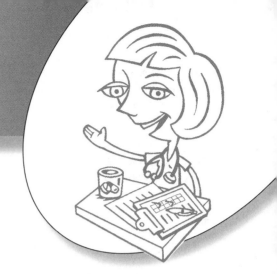

Note: Page numbers followed by *f* or *t* indicate figures or tables, respectively.